GET
HEALTHY

LIVE
LEAN

LOVE YOUR BODY

The Real Secret to Weight Loss and Lifetime Fitness

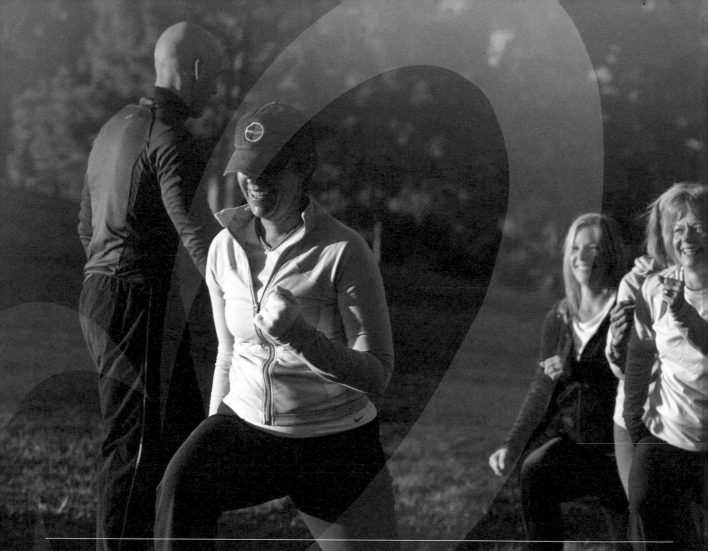

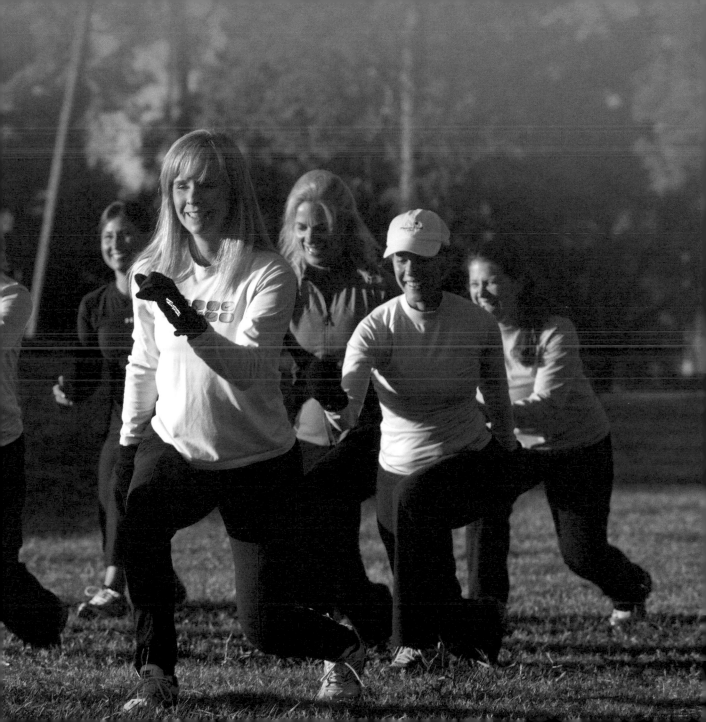

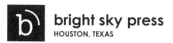

bright sky press
HOUSTON, TEXAS

2365 Rice Boulevard, Suite 202,
Houston, Texas 77005

10   9   8   7   6   5   4   3   2   1

Library of Congress Cataloging-in-Publication Data

Hughes, Bethany.
Love your body : the real secret to weight loss & lifetime fitness / from the founders of
Love Your Body Fitness boot camps Bethany Hughes and Vince Grbic.
p. cm.
ISBN 978-1-933979-61-8 (softcover with flaps : alk. paper)
1. Physical fitness. 2. Exercise. 3. Weight loss. I. Grbic, Vince. II. Title.

GV481.H779 2009
613.7--dc22   2009010067

Book and cover design by Cregan Design, Marla Garcia
Photography by Michael Hart, with photo on page 16 by Cindy Cady.
Edited by Nora Shire.
Printed in the U.S.A. at RRDonnelley

ACKNOWLEDGMENTS

I wrote this book for my children, Haddon and Parker, so that they would know the secrets to living lean from the beginning. I hope they stay healthy and as active as they are now! Haddon, you will never let me get by with anything, and your dedication to your endeavors inspires me every day! You are a joy. Parker, your sense of humor keeps our family laughing, and your sharp wit and your kind heart never let us down. I have to stay on my toes to keep up with you. I would like to thank my husband, Jim, for suggesting I start strength training in the first place. I couldn't have done this without your support, help with the kids in the mornings and your great cooking!

To my Mom and Dad, the most supportive parents anyone could ask for. Thank you for all you have done for me throughout my entire life. Thank you Aunt Mimi for reading the book and helping edit it. You, too, have been there for me my whole life.

To the women I have worked out with — you have made this past few years so much fun. I cannot thank you enough for pushing me and inspiring me. You all are amazing! I have learned so much from all of you. I also appreciate the "fitness models" in this book — you know who you are! Thanks to my first group of friends who did Hill Runs with me at the park and believed that sprinting really is fun! Also my T/Th group — and that includes our evenings out as well!

We also want to thank One to One for allowing us to take photos in their wonderful gym — the blonde Brigade loves you Todd!

I couldn't have written this book without Lucy Chambers. She gave my words the spark that I could never have imparted. She is my voice, and I could never have done this without her encouragement. Ellen Cregan and Marla Garcia are an amazing and creative design team. Michael Hart, your photography was amazing and thanks for all the extra time!

I thank Jim Guillory, my Muscle Activation Technique specialist for keeping my body in working order. When things shut down, he is there to make me feel 20 again! I would also like to thank the Houston Parks and Recreation Department for keeping the parks a lovely place to exercise.

Thank you Tom McCaffrey and Tim Horan — our lawyers, Monty Allen and Tracy, our accountants, Chris Gerow, our banker, Tricia Bell who is keeping us on task, and Mark Woodruff, who has helped with our website and been our sounding board.

Finally, I thank my friend, business partner, and trainer, Vince Grbic. It was his never-ending encouragement that gave me the confidence to change my life. He made it fun, simple and easy to get fit. He also kept it fresh and continues to challenge me. His energy and his positive outlook make me wish that he could train every woman. For those who think they are stuck as a size 14 or more, let me tell you, you CAN DO IT — it isn't too late to change your life and do all that you want to do!

— Bethany Hughes

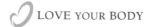

ACKNOWLEDGMENTS

First, I want to thank my wife, Kathleen, for all her support through all my long nights in front of the computer and my constant early risings. She became chauffeur to our youngest and sometimes secretary to me.

I want to thank my children, Kirstin and Ashton for the love and support they provide me, even when I am an often an absent dad. I wrote this book with them in mind. I want them to have the knowledge to keep them healthy and strong throughout their lives.

None of this would have come together without Bright Sky Press. Lucy, Ellen and the whole staff are smart and accommodating and make me sound better than I could have imagined!

Thanks to Michael Hart for the brilliant photos. He is an artist behind the lens.

I want to thank one of my best friends, Mark Woodruff, for his advice and making our web site look great.

I want to thank my parents for their love and support.

Thanks to our trainers Blake Williamson and Daniel Oliver. Their commitment to giving our clients a fun, safe and memorable experience has truly kept Love Your Body Fitness Boot Camps going.

I want to thank the staff of what I consider to be one of the greatest fitness clubs in the country, The Houstonian Hotel, Club and Spa. Their dedication to the membership is legendary and inspiring. I have been privileged to work next to some of the most innovative and energetic trainers for almost ten years, and I learn from them daily.

There is one person who has made this all happen. Without her, I would not be doing this. Bethany Hughes has been a friend and inspiration to me since I met her over three years ago. When we started training together, I never would have imagined we would start a business, write a book and strive to give women a place to gather information that will help them feel great! She is driven to help people achieve their wellness goals, and she is a driving force in our business.

— Vince Grbic

DEDICATIONS

To our hardworking boot campers who have inspired
us to share our message with others

TABLE OF CONTENTS

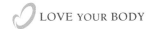
TESTIMONIALS

I JOINED LOVE YOUR BODY FITNESS WITH A FRIEND, NEVER ANTICIPATING THAT I WOULD MAKE NEW FRIENDS OR ENJOY WORKING OUT SO MUCH. It had been a while (maybe a long while) since I had exercised, but I quickly lost inches and weight as we moved from one adventure to the next. I love the sense of camaraderie and accomplishment that comes with each class. The other "campers" encourage one another to "go for it" but without a sense of competitiveness. Best of all, now I am wearing clothes that had been sitting in my closet (like long-lost friends) and having fun at the same time. What a great feeling — losing weight with friends while playing.

Bethany was truly inspirational showing me what was possible to accomplish with my own fitness. She never lectures or makes us feel "bad" about where we are in the fitness process and truly meets you where you are and inspires you to go further than you think possible. Mostly, she makes the impossible obtainable. Her message is a real life "success story," and I still look at her story, which is a path I want to follow.

I would encourage everyone to join the boot camp program or read the book to understand what the approach is all about. There is room for everyone in Love Your Body — from beginner to the world-class athlete. Come join the fun and learn how to love yourself.

– Lisa Hall
Attorney/Consultant

AT THE END OF 1997 I HAD BYPASS SURGERY. The day following the operation, I had a massive heart attack which put me in the cardiac intensive care unit for forty days. Despite this great damage to my heart, I have lived a full life these past 10 years. Now, a new aortic valve gives me the opportunity for more.

When I began my recovery ten years ago, I understood my survival depended on three important areas — diet, medications and exercise. I have taken my medications faithfully, but I only deserve an average grade for diet. If I have made up for that in any way, it has been my dedication to exercise.

As founder of Academy Sports & Outdoors, I should know something about exercise. I don't. Vince Grbic has been my trainer. I totally depended on Vince to show me what to do.

After my aortic valve replacement, my family was told that the surgery was less difficult than expected because, despite the permanent damage my heart sustained in 1997, I am in good physical condition.

For that, I thank Vince. His skills as a trainer have given me more than 10 good years.

– Arthur Gochman
Founder of Academy Sports and Outdoors

8

FOREWORD

The statistics are staggering: According to data from the National Health and Nutrition Examination Survey (NHANES) 2001-2004, two-thirds of adults in the U.S. are overweight. The next time you're at a soccer game or walking through the mall, look around: Two out of every three adults are obese, out of shape, and at serious risk of diabetes, heart disease, stroke, osteoarthritis, and some types of cancer.[1]

The bad news is we're getting fatter: From 1960 to 2004, the prevalence of overweight increased from just under 50% to the current two-thirds of adults. Almost 60% of adults get absolutely no exercise.[1] How much do you want to bet that these are the same folks who are overweight?

More bad news: The research is clear that dieting just doesn't work. An analysis of 31 long-term dieting studies shows just what we already know from personal experience: Two to five years after losing weight, the majority of people regained all the weight they lost; 30-60% of those people actually gained more weight than they lost.[2]

Now here's the good news: Love Your Body Fitness. I've been a nutrition and health professional for almost 20 years, and Love Your Body Fitness is a breath of fresh air. Vince and Bethany's message is absolutely critical: When we love our bodies, engage in fun and well-planned exercise, and choose healthy foods, we feel great, increase our energy levels, and lose weight. We don't need to diet to lose weight. Instead of a diet, Vince and Bethany use common sense, practical tips on changing our eating and activity habits in a lifestyle approach.

How is a lifestyle approach different from a diet? It puts you in charge. It is not a diet book or counselor, or printed diet from the Web. You decide to eat frequently throughout the day, choosing healthy foods in moderate portions. You decide how often you want to eat out, and make choices about the types of foods you truly want to eat. It's up to you to plan exercise into your day and make it as much a part of your routine as brushing your teeth. Most important is this simple statement: You love your body instead of hating it. Once we truly decide to love our body, lumps and all, everything else falls into place.

Of course you don't have to do all of this by yourself. This book outlines everything you need to know, gives you practical tips and makes suggestions. The authors tell you how to implement changes in eating habits and activities to help you lose weight, increase strength, and feel great about yourself. Helpful tools including a food journal, protein sources with portion information, and specific exercise instructions help you make simple changes in your lifestyle to reach your goals.

One of my favorite aspects of this book is the focus on loving your body and setting goals that are realistic, obtainable, and meaningful to you. All too often we decide to lose weight or get in shape for someone else: our doctor, our spouse, our friends. Bethany and Vince demand that you focus on yourself and the goals that are important to you. Without this emphasis on putting yourself first, you're simply not going to succeed. Love Your Body isn't a diet plan, it's a blueprint for empowering women to take charge of our lives and our bodies.

9

Three years ago my sister started taking Vince and Bethany's boot camp classes, raving all the time about the energy and fun she had before the sun came up on a Saturday morning. Two years ago I visited my sister in Houston, and she insisted I take a Boot Camp class with her. Again, it was before sunrise on a Saturday morning. I had a blast!

I felt like a little kid running around the playground again, having a ball with my new-found friends, and often pushing that same 8-pound ball over my head while jogging around a fitness path, followed by lots of skipping and jumping. There was no yelling, just lots of laughter. No shouting, just tons of encouragement. Vince and Bethany have captured that same fun by encouraging a we're-all-in-this-together attitude in their book. They will inspire you to start loving your body, even if you decide to skip the sunrise exercise time.

Lynn Grieger, RD, CDE
Health, Food and Fitness coach
Manchester, VT
www.LynnGrieger.com

10

---

[1] Statistics Related to Overweight and Obesity, Weight-control Information Network, May 2007. Accessed 9-15-08 at http://win.niddk.nih.gov/statistics

[2] Mann T et al (2007), Medicare's search for effective obesity treatments: diets are not the answer. American Psychologist Vol 62, issue 3; pg 220-233.

Introduction

You picked up this book because you want to be in shape — and who doesn't? But if you are anything like us, you've tried lots of routines and diets that may have worked for a while, but when life got in the way, you slid back into your old habits, your old fitness level, and your old clothes.

We know where you are, because we were there, and as frustrated as you are. We founded Love Your Body Fitness — no yelling, go-at-your-own-pace boot camps for women — so that you won't have to spend another day frustrated with your body, believing that you have no control over it. Along with our exercise programs, we have developed a personalized approach to combining nutrition with fitness. It is based on who you are and the constraints of your crazy busy life so you can get up, get to the gym, and get in shape — for good, this time!

Before we discovered the information we will share with you, we were an out-of-shape personal trainer and a frazzled carpool mom. We were always wondering why we didn't have enough energy to do what we wanted to do, why our backs were bothering us all the time, and why we never felt satisfied with our physical selves.

Once we started consciously making the choices to love our bodies, we knew we were on to something so powerful and so attainable we had to share it with everyone we know. In 2006, we founded Love Your Body Fitness Boot Camps, so that anyone who wants to can have a strong healthy body. And even more importantly, a body that is filled with energy and joy!

Making the choice to love our bodies — to finally accept who we are and what works for us — has changed our bodies, our attitudes, and our lives. Take a little time to read our fitness and nutrition guidelines and see if our fitness journeys don't sound familiar to you. Not only can we help you be your own personal trainer, but we can help you look like one, too.

Bethany　　*Vince*

BETHANY'S STORY

In January 2005 I had a pair of black pants, size 14. They were the only pants in my closet that fit. For an entire winter I changed the shoes and jackets but always had on those black pants. On off-days I wore sweats. I was in denial. I told myself that I just wasn't as hung up on clothes as some of my friends. Noble causes filled my hours — taking care of my kids and being an active volunteer. Then, one day, I decided to see what I weighed. It couldn't be that bad. I jumped on the scale and to my dismay I weighed only two pounds less than when I was about to deliver my babies.

Disgusted and depressed, I realized I had to do something. Even if I didn't care about clothes, I cared about my husband and my children. I wanted to feel better and get healthy. I had so much experience (and so many failures) with crash diets and low-carb planned programs, that I knew I needed something completely different. Not a diet, but a new lifestyle, one that I could maintain forever. I started my search. There was so much information online and in magazines that it was confusing and hard for me to put it all together in a sensible way. So I just slowly started muddling through all the information.

13

The first step was eating differently and exercising. The second step was inviting friends to join me for walks and exercise sessions as I began to lose weight and firm up. Before I found the combination of diet and exercise that brought me to this point of really loving my body, I went through much trial and error. I just wish I had known 20 years ago what I know now. What fun I could have had! I am now a size 4. The number doesn't matter, except that it is the right size for my frame and musculature. What does matter is that it feels fantastic to be lean and strong.

I'm sharing my story with you so you'll understand how much power these habits have in changing your relationship with your body. No matter how close you are to giving up ever feeling good about your body, you'll see that there is hope. If I can love my body like I do now, you can, too.

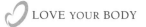

BEGINNING LOVE YOUR BODY FITNESS

After a lifetime of battling weight, in September of 2005 I started working out with Vince. Through my own trial and error, I had found some diet and exercise strategies that were starting to show results, but I could tell that other important pieces were missing. Once Vince and I put our heads together, I found the program I had been looking for my whole life.

One of my four workouts each week was a boot camp-style activity. When the indoor basketball court became confining for me, I asked Vince if we could take the workout outdoors. We began to train at one of the public parks in Houston. It had a large hill and a running track. It was winter, often cold, and I felt like Vince was torturing me! Eight weeks later, I realized that he was on to something, and that with friends to share my "misery," it might even be fun. Vince said he'd be happy to accommodate a group, so I e-mailed about 20 of my closest friends and invited them to join me.

Almost immediately 10 said yes, and soon we had a wait list of three. With my encouragement Vince got a second trainer. I went to work e-mailing a larger group of friends, and we started "Babe-a-licious" Boot Camp. For two months, we giggled, laughed, and huffed and puffed our way around the park. Summer was coming, and we decided we wanted a second class. We added a Wednesday morning session to the Saturday class and began offering the program twice a week.

Throughout the hot Houston summer, these women were actually having fun. Many began to see results for the first time ever. Some of the original boot campers have continued and are with us today! Fall came, and I suggested a 9 a.m. class for those with small kids and 8:30 a.m. drop-offs. Vince was able to teach the class, and again, just by e-mailing my buddies, it filled up.

Slowly we added other classes, and I had to learn Excel. About this time Vince suggested that we were on to something big, and I should consider making Boot Camp my full-time job. After several months, I agreed. I quit my job as an art consultant, and we formed a partnership. Since then, the classes have grown — friends of friends have come in. I am constantly meeting new women who all share in the same frustration with their current approach to fitness and the same desire for a pleasurable way to get in shape and stay there. I am always amazed at how small a world it really is! We have had "grandmothers" and "little sisters" come to Boot Camp. Today, the age range is basically 28 to 60, but I'm always hoping that a 70-year-old will join! What Vince showed me — and we have seen validated in the lives of hundreds of women — is that Boot Camp coupled with good nutrition is the key to a fit and toned body. Read on, and we'll share all the secrets of Love Your Body Boot Camp.

MAKING IT A COMMUNITY

Once the boot camps were under way, we realized we were experiencing something important. Friends who never wanted to exercise and women, who previously could only exercise with a personal trainer breathing down their necks, were suddenly coming out at sunrise on Saturday mornings to sweat and laugh together. What seemed so painful to do alone was actually fun with friends. Women told us that all the inertia of getting off the couch and putting on those athletic shoes fizzled away when they thought about coming out to join us.

Sure, there was trepidation before their first time, but once they experienced the camaraderie of our boot camp, they began to look forward to exercising. Like a book club, a lunch date, or a long cup of coffee with a friend, boot camp was a social time. Watching other women puff and grunt and smile and laugh made everyone realize that getting or staying in shape was a challenge for everybody. There wasn't anybody out there who had a body that automatically kept itself fit all the time. We were all in this together.

So what worked? What was the big draw that kept women coming back for more, telling their friends, and feeling great? Community: Women of all shapes and sizes, all sharing the same goal of being fit and feeling good. Women wanted a positive atmosphere when they exercised, not a drill sergeant barking at them. These women wanted to be recognized as real, warm bodies, not disembodied e-mails or blog posts. The physical togetherness was an important part of the powerfully positive experience everyone was having at Boot Camp.

As our world spins faster and faster, and women work harder than ever at taking care of their families and their jobs, time to interact with friends becomes more limited and more precious. Dedicating an hour or more to feeling physically strong and being with others — not just alone on a track or in a gym full of strangers with a paid companion — becomes truly meaningful. Boot camp brought us together, and the togetherness cemented our motivation to become fit and our determination to help each other reach that goal.

REALIZING YOU CAN'T DO IT ALONE

Love Your Body Fitness Boot Camp. We thought long and hard before we named our camps. Each of those words is important. Love: We know personally that you're going to love how you feel when focusing on fitness rather than food. Your: It's your body, not anybody else's. No one else knows what makes you feel good from the inside out more than you. Body: That's what it's all about. Getting that body moving, feeding that body what it needs. Fitness: This is what makes it all happen. Boot: And yes, you're going to have to put a little power into it. Boot it up! But it's the Camp part of the formula that makes it so successful: You don't need to do it alone.

Read on. Learn what we do at boot camp. Find out how really out of shape we were before we learned what we know now. Find out what our secrets are. You'll see that most of them aren't really secret, they're just tried and true fitness and nutrition tips. It's no secret that to get fit you eat less and exercise more. But just how do you accomplish that? How much less do you eat of what? How much more of what kind of exercise do you do? We've sorted through the overwhelming multitude of diets and workout plans and organized them in the most accessible way possible so you can get what you need to get going.

Once you understand what to do, find your fellow campers and get to work. You might have a few friends from work, a neighbor, or even a whole bunch of buddies who want to get in shape — their own best shape — together. And we're here to support you — at our camps and online. Once you say out loud, "I want to love my body," you'll be amazed how many others want to join you on your journey. It's a team thing, and there's no yelling.

BETHANY
BEFORE & AFTER

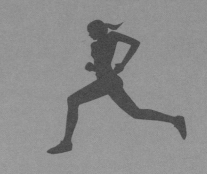

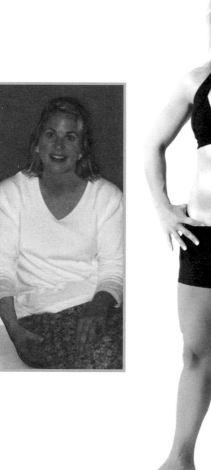

WHY WEIGHT?

"How did I lose my weight? I sweat hard. I eat well. I listen to my body. I keep moving seven days a week. I may choose an easy workout if I have pushed myself hard for a couple of days, but I always keep it fun and challenging. Now that I love my body, I do strength training three days each week, and I do cardio on average six to seven days a week. But I started out slowly and worked up to this.

Keeping it fun is the key. I always listen to new music. When I first wanted to get in shape, it was so lonely. I felt like I was the only person I knew who had a weight problem. But then I made friends at the gym. Now I've made so many friends through my gym and the boot camps that I can't wait to exercise. If you had told me I would be disappointed to miss a workout, I would have laughed. If you had told me that I would convince all my friends to get up early on a Saturday to do boot camp together, I would have laughed out loud.

The eating and exercise tips that Vince and I are going to share with you in this book have changed my life, and I have never been happier.

You can love your body, too. Why weight?"

VINCE
BEFORE & AFTER

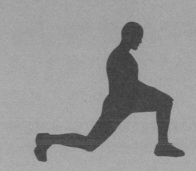

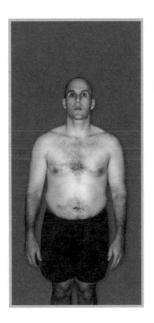

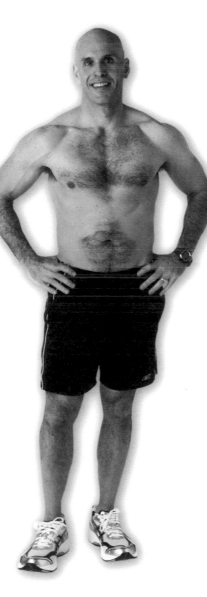

GET MOVING!

"Here's the bottom line: Eat fewer calories than you burn. We are much less active than we were even 10 years ago. Gyms are plentiful and want your business, so you can get a good deal on a membership. If you don't like gyms, try walking to work, parking farther away, taking the stairs or doing your own lawn. If just two weeks of inactivity can start packing on abdominal fat, there's no time to lose. Think back about the last time you really exercised on a regular basis and you'll realize how important it is to get moving. Remember, it really doesn't matter how — Just move!"

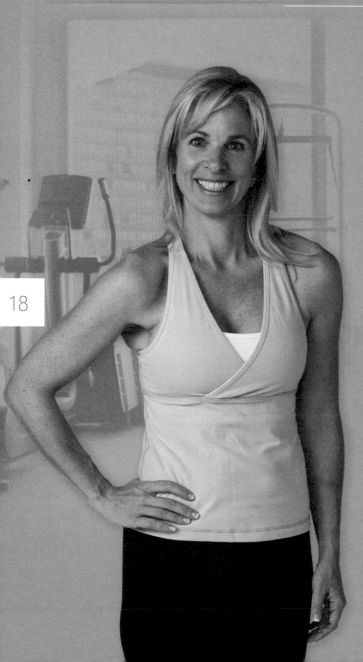

18

I never considered myself fat as a child, but my life revolved around food. I was always thinking about my next meal or snack. I didn't think about nutrition. I ate whatever I thought sounded good at the time, and always ate until I didn't have room for one more bite. I knew my mom would always give in if I pushed hard enough. In the 5th grade, I was the tallest in my class and weighted 83 pounds. All I wanted was to weigh 65 pounds like all my buddies!

By 8th grade I realized that I was overweight, and I embarked on the first of many diets I would fail for the next 35 years. The diet I chose lasted two weeks and spelled out what to eat for every meal. I lost some weight, but I gained it right back because I hated being told what to do.

All those diets were about rules and numbers and how much you weighed. Now I know that the numbers mean nothing. It's really about fitness and health and body-fat ratio. Sure that's a number, but it's your own number based on your height, frame and musculature.

Everyone dreams of going to college and making a fresh start. Even after a summer of fierce dieting, I was still on the medium to heavy side. In college I ate the usual — pizza at midnight, popcorn and Mexican food. I resorted to camouflage — long skirts with grosgrain ribbon belts and oxford cloth shirts. I could not deprive myself of anything and it really showed. This attitude continued into my marriage.

When my husband took a job in Houston in April 1994, I was back to a size 14. I had two children 17 months apart and had worked up to 177 pounds. I told myself my husband loved me for who I was.

Then I reached my 40th birthday and still weighed 177 pounds. I thought "I CANNOT BE FAT AND 40!" I went on a severe diet that cut out all sugar, and I lost about 15 pounds. Within two years, I was right back up there. Yikes! I spent one afternoon sobbing my heart out, and the next day I bought a pair of running shoes. I hauled my big ol' self out to that park and hoofed around the trail. I could barely run/walk two miles. Again and again I went out running, not knowing what else to do, and desperately wanting to escape from the body I found myself trapped in.

Realizing I needed a diet for life, I began asking my trim and fit friends what they ate. They all had useful tips that had helped them find a way of eating that worked for their body type. I learned a lot: Eating Greek yogurt would up the protein in my diet; having another meal during the day would help me eat less; and having a healthy shake at 4 p.m. would give me energy and keep me from snacking.

Another friend recommended *Body For Life for Women*. It gave me even more motivation.

I continued to run and started to rollerblade. I lost about 15 pounds, and there was no diet in sight. I was not watching my food intake. The loss was all from the exercise. My kids were getting older, and I had the time to think about my nutrition and focus again on myself. Being healthy so I could be around for them longer became truly important to me.

For the first time in my life I began to care about what I ate. By adding more fruits and vegetables plus lean meats, I started feeling better. When I upped the protein, I had more energy and was satisfied. The weight loss continued. It was a by-product of the good choices I was making. There was no deprivation.

At the gym, I began with the elliptical trainer and pushed myself to go longer each time. I also began lifting weights. That afternoon I spent crying, I weighed 175 pounds, and I couldn't find any jeans that fit. I nervously went to the Gap and found a pair of 12s I could squeeze into. Two months later I had to buy a pair of 10s, and three months after that the 8 fit. It felt amazing that all of me could fit into those little jeans. It didn't stop there. I now wear a 2.

My husband could tell how energized and happy I was to be taking care of myself. He suggested that I hire a personal trainer who could teach me safe and effective ways to lose fat and gain muscle and not focus on the number on the scale.

Training with Vince Grbic began my understanding of weight plus body fat vs. muscle. He showed me how to use a combination of free weights and machines in a safe and balanced way. My lower back had been bothering me for years, but as I strengthened my core I had no more issues. I was amazed at how my body began to change, going from 155 lbs to 135 in 6 months. After teaching me how to use other cardio machines, Vince asked me to start keeping a food diary. He had me walking at an incline on the treadmill. I have never perspired so much or worked so hard, but I loved it!

When I began to train, my body was over 30 percent fat, and this was after losing 20 pounds! Lifting weights brought it down to 19 percent. My optimal range should be 17-27 percent. Now I exercise enough that I can eat "off-limits" foods when I want them. By adding weight training to my cardio and good nutrition I had finally found the key to loving my body! The combination made all the difference for me, and it will for you, too.

VINCE'S STORY

I may be a personal trainer now, and you might find this hard to believe, but I've had to battle my weight my whole life. I was always a chunky kid. I grew up on sugar and butter sandwiches, chicken- fried steak and McDonald's. Even though I was athletic and excelled at sports, I ate anything that was served. My big three staples were pizza, hamburgers and fried chicken. My father came from South America in 1959. He loved all the new restaurants, especially fast food. My brother and I developed a taste for it early. A balanced meal was a hamburger and French fries — meat, dairy (cheese) and vegetable (potato). No wonder I always felt fat. I remember slugging someone in junior high for berating me about my weight. By my freshman year in high school, I had had enough.

My mother had started a popular diet program. I followed what she ate and did what she did, and I lost weight too. I cut portions, stopped eating fried foods, and I did a food diary. By the summer before 10th grade, I had lost about 20 pounds. It made all the difference. Girls began to notice me for the first time ever. I stayed active in sports throughout high school and continued to eat fairly well. I was determined that I would never be fat again.

I still felt fat inside though. Because of so much exercise, I often injured myself. I had two back surgeries and one knee surgery. I wish I had felt better about myself so that I wouldn't have strived for perfection. Running wasn't good enough unless I could run for an hour. If I just had a little window of time, I wouldn't even go. It wasn't worth it to run for 30 minutes — it wasn't good enough. Weight training and cardiovascular exercise came easy for me. I worked at all the gyms in college and went on to become a personal trainer.

Nutrition remained my Achilles heel. I knew healthy eating was the key. I had gone to graduate school to get my master's in education, health and exercise-related fitness, but I wouldn't take the next step. I spent my 30s going up and down in weight. Becoming discouraged, I lost my motivation along the way. I became complacent and had a 36-inch waist and a spare tire. Middle age had arrived. I made excuse after excuse. Finishing my kid's meals and eating what I wanted, all because I thought it was satisfying me. So why didn't I feel good?

In the fall of 2005, my body fat was over 20%. As a personal trainer, I knew that was not acceptable. Both my health and job were in jeopardy. Shocked that my body fat had gotten so high, I finally made the decision to practice what I had been telling my clients all along. No surprise, I began to lose the weight.

We have software at my gym that will give a body's age based on physical assessments like body fat, strength and cardiovascular fitness. I challenged Bethany to a body age contest. Although we were both well into our 40s, this program revealed that by loving our bodies three ways — cardio, resistance training, and nutrition — her body age was 29 and mine was 30!

We knew we were on to something too good to keep to ourselves.

WHAT'S YOUR MOTIVATION?

People who have lost weight and kept it off say that their primary goal was to get healthy, not to lose weight. Weight loss is a by-product of lowering your cholesterol and blood pressure and simply working to feel better and have more energy. In order to be successful at any endeavor, you have to set a goal. Getting fit is no different. There are many aspects to getting fit, and you are the only one who knows what you want and need. Do you want more energy? Do you want to look more attractive? Do you want to be stronger? Do you want to be healthier? Those are big goals, and there are not many people out there who wouldn't like to attain them, if they are honest with themselves. But there are other goals, too.

Do you want to fit into a special dress you have for a party? Are you getting married? Are you turning 30, or 40, or 50, and you just can't face it without feeling your best? Do you want to look hot for your husband, boyfriend, or date? Are you going on a hiking or biking trip and you're nervous that it will be difficult because you are out of shape? The list goes on, and there is no bad motivation. The important thing is to set goals and remain motivated to reach them.

What do you want to accomplish? How often will you check in? What's going to keep you motivated? Write it down, and refer to it often.

My clients can tell me much more about their bodies than I can tell them. I want them to be in touch with how they feel, when they hurt and when they are tired. I tell them that my biggest concern is that they have a safe and fun workout. We change exercises, number of reps, and exercise intensity. I explain to them that their bodies

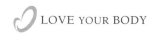
will become too efficient if they do the same thing over and over again. Changing things up causes their bodies to continue to adapt, and that means more strength and cardiovascular endurance.

I hear people say that they can't strength train until they lose weight. This is backwards thinking. Strength training helps you lose weight. Lean muscle burns more efficiently and is heavier, and therefore burns more calories! The most effective way to stay healthy is to eat properly, strength train and move your body.

SETTING LONG-TERM GOALS AND SHORT-TERM GOALS

Starting to waffle? Read on! Our short-term goal is to convince you that you can have the body that you were meant to have. Our long-term goal is to show you how to do it and keep you motivated. You're going to love it!

The most effective way to stay healthy is to eat properly, strength train and move your body.

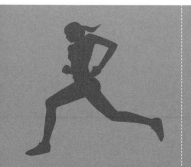

BEFORE YOU SET YOUR GOALS, THINK ABOUT WHO YOU REALLY ARE AND WHAT YOU REALLY WANT. Think about really attractive people with your frame. Look around you. Realize that stunning healthy women come in all sizes. Don't compare yourself to people who are built completely different from you. Then think about your own body. What do you like about it? What do you want to work on? Are your arms flabby? Does your stomach pooch out? Do you want more muscle tone in your legs? Dropping excess fat and toning your body will help all around, but identify the areas where you want to see specific improvement.

Chapter 1

Are You Ready to Love Your Body?

ADMIT IT, YOU'RE OUT OF SHAPE

The signs are there, and they're undeniable: You look at your backside in the mirror, and the shelf around your waist looks more like a middle-aged mother-in-law than a cute young mom. You try to convince yourself that you're just solid, but there's no getting around it — you've gotten frumpy. If you poke your stomach out really far, you can actually look pregnant — full-term, not first trimester. You have to stand up really straight and make sure that you don't lift your arms too high, or the dewlaps over your bra are downright disgusting. And your poor arms look like they belong to a flying squirrel.

And we won't mention your clothes. They are crying out to get your attention: Your most comfortable jeans are tight around the waist — all the time, not only when they're just out of the dryer. You find yourself wanting to get out of those work clothes as fast as possible and into comfy sweats, because the more fitted clothes irritate you. You spend more time putting on makeup and jewelry and choosing outfits, because you don't feel like you look good anymore unless everything is perfect.

Then there are your muscles: Reaching back to get one of the kids to settle down in the car, and your neck goes into death lock. You see a friend at a restaurant, turning in your seat to give him a kiss, and a knife shoots through your lower back. Your calves are cramping in your high heels, and, mainly, you're just downright tired.

Some days you rationalize that you're just not as young as before. Other days, after a good night's sleep and you're just around old friends who love you "no matter what," you don't think about it. The day before your period when everything seems terrible, you feel like your body has completely betrayed you. Since there's nothing you can do about it, you might as well hit the Oreos hard and start again tomorrow.

But the truth is, you're not old, fat, or hopeless: You are just out of shape, and you can fix it.

How did you get this way? You might not know. Maybe you were captain of the tennis team in high school and still play on a team. Maybe you jog every day (well, almost every day). Maybe you lost 15 pounds doing South Beach two years ago, you're still not eating much, and you don't know why you just feel dumpier and dumpier. Or you might have a pretty good idea. Maybe you never lost the baby

But the truth is, you're not old, fat, or hopeless: you're just out of shape, and you can fix it.

25

fat from your first child before you had the second. Maybe those chicken tenders that your little girl leaves on her plate are too tempting to pass up. Maybe calories eaten standing up really do count. Maybe you were just meant to be a heavy person and you should quit fighting it and be thankful for all your blessings.

Stop! It doesn't matter how you got out of shape. Life hits all of us with an infinite variety of complications and challenges, and our bodies just want to help us feel better. They tell us, wouldn't a cookie taste good now? Or, I think a glass of wine might take the edge off here. But luckily, we don't have to listen. We can make our bodies feel better, and look better, and have more energy without going to a spa, or going on the wagon, or being miserable. We can live our busy lives, meet the needs of our husbands, boyfriends, children, parents, and — most importantly — ourselves, and still be fit and feel great.

Ha, you say. Everyone you know who looks great has a nanny to keep her kids while she works out with a personal trainer, or doesn't work, or has good genes. Fitness may work for those women, but I don't have time for it right now. Well, we hate to burst the bubble of illusions that has been keeping you down-and-out-of-shape, but we know you can do it — no matter what your situation is with your babysitters, your work, or your genes. In fact, we're going to go so far as to say we can teach you how to take your family out for Mexican food, go out with your book club, attend as many parties as your work or PTA demands, and still look buff and feel babe-a-licious.

GET BUFF, FEEL BABE-A-LICIOUS

Buff? Babe-a-licious? What do we mean? Buff means just having good muscle tone, being physically fit and trim. It doesn't mean you stand in front of the mirror at the gym and admire your oiled "six-pack" abdominal muscles. And babe-a-licious doesn't mean you need to get a navel ring and go around showing more skin than your grandmother would approve of. It means being a woman who is highly pleasing to the senses. A young-at-heart woman who takes care of her body, lives a healthy lifestyle, fits in her own clothes comfortably, and meets the world with confidence — whether or not she has time to put on a jacket that covers her hips.

No matter what your chronological age is, you can be that buff young woman who is babe-a-licious. Having all the energy needed to meet the demands of your life. You can fit into your skinniest jeans — not your neighbor's, not your sister's, but yours — and maybe even a smaller size. But most importantly, making friends with your body

means working with it instead of beating it up in the gym or starving it into submission. You can start loving your body today.

HOW DO YOU DO IT?

We're going to tell you specifically what to do to get your nutrition and exercise in order to be fit and healthy. But we can't do it for you. Before reading any further, admit to yourself you are sick and tired (perhaps even literally) of not feeling and looking your best. You have to say out loud, "I'm getting back in shape." Say it a few times — to your best friend, your mother, your husband, your supportive coworker. Write it on a little sticky note and put it on your bathroom mirror. Put another one on your refrigerator. Now believe it. Even if you don't believe it yet, say it like you believe it. Act like you believe it. And believe it or not, before you know it, it will come true.

We're not saying that you won't have setbacks along the way. We're not saying that you won't have days when you feel frumpy or blue. But before getting started, it is important that you know big dreams eclipse setbacks. Whether or not you really believe deep down that you want to get fit, you do. Whether or not you really believe that you can do it, you can. There is not a rationalization you can come up with that we haven't wrestled with when we were out-of-shape. We know just how daunting it is to take those first few steps toward committing to make a change. But we also know that if we can do it, if all the women who have successfully come through our boot camps can do it, you can do it. So no ifs or buts or whens; it's agreed. You are getting in shape. And when you feel good from the inside out, you will thank yourself for it.

READY OR NOT, HERE YOU GO!

First, you need to ask yourself some questions. Find a quiet minute to focus — before you go to bed, or set your alarm a few minutes earlier than usual. Think about your current level of frustration with your body and ask yourself honestly what your goals are. Do you need more energy? Do you need to lower your blood pressure or cholesterol? Do you just want to be stronger and healthier? Is the goal to fit into your own clothes again, or into new, smaller clothes? Do you want to lose weight?

Once you determine your goals, write them down. You don't need to journal extensively. Even little Post-Its can keep you focused. Don't judge your goals — just like we all have different bodies, we all have different desires for them. If you have a beautiful dress that you'd like to wear to a Christmas party, and getting it zipped motivates you to learn to love your body, it is just as valid and important a reason to get fit as wanting to have more energy to support your family. Your reasons are your own, and your new buff self will benefit every area of your life, no matter what motivated you to get that way.

Now, answer the following questions:

1. Does your doctor say that you can start working out?
2. Are you willing to exercise more often?
3. Are you willing to add more hours of rest each night so that you get a good night's sleep?
4. Are you willing to get up early to work out?
5. Are you willing to keep a food diary?
6. Are you willing to cut down on alcohol and/or cut calorie intake?
7. If you have extra stress in your life, can you make a change or get help to reduce it?

The answer to all of these questions must be yes. If you answered no to any of them, ask yourself why. "I tried before, and I couldn't do it" isn't an acceptable answer. Remember, just as it doesn't matter how you got out of shape, it doesn't matter what you have tried to do before to get in shape. What does matter — what is non-negotiable — is that you believe that you are getting in shape now. If you don't quite believe it yet, look at those little sticky notes you put up, say "I'm getting in shape," and fake it until you make it.

GOOD GOALS ARE OBTAINABLE

Goals are not like gifts from fairy godmothers that just appear when we are especially deserving. Goals are ideals that we set for ourselves and systematically move towards achieving. Other people cannot set real goals for us — they can only challenge us. If you want to get in shape because you think your husband would love you more, your real goal isn't getting in shape, it's getting closer to your husband. If you want to be leaner because you feel awkward around all your fit friends, your goal isn't losing weight, it's being comfortable around your friends.

It's important to know why you are setting the goals you desire, and it's important that you set them only for yourself. Sure, there will be fringe benefits all around — you will get a response from your husband and feel more comfortable stepping out with your friends, we guarantee it — but you won't stay buff unless you get that way for yourself.

If you think others might motivate the goals you set, go back and look at them again. Don't be afraid to say you

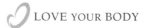

want to look and feel great just for you. Don't fall into the Good Woman trap of putting everyone else first — if you truly want to do a good job of being responsible for your family, take care of yourself first. Being tired and unhealthy doesn't do anybody any good, and it does not make you a good role model.

Once your own goals are identified, break them down into steps. You want to lose 10 pounds? Great. What will you do each week to get there? How fast can you go, realistically, and stay healthy? You want more energy? That's less tangible, but start noticing how you feel when you get up in the morning and when you go to bed. Do you have a lull in the afternoon when you just want to lie down on the couch and shut your eyes for a minute? Jot that down now, and once a week look at those questions. By writing down the new or updated answers, you can track your progress towards that big goal in the short term.

Do you have bad eating habits? Choose one aspect of your diet to improve each week, and get healthier step by step. Meeting short-term goals, one at a time, will keep you headed for the big prize and keep you from getting overwhelmed or dejected along the way. If you slip up on your short-term goal, you're not offtrack. Just start right over where you left off, and you are still headed toward success.

WHAT LOVING YOUR BODY REALLY MEANS

As you set goals, remember that loving your body doesn't mean Vogue magazine will call you up to be on the cover. It doesn't mean that your nose will suddenly look perfect, or that everyone will draw their breath when you walk into the room. It means you have made a promise to yourself to respect and be responsible for your one and only body. And that you will take care of it until death do you part. You will honor it by appreciating its strengths, acknowledging its weaknesses, and working with both so that you can feel as comfortable and happy as possible in it. It means that you will not eat a basketful of chips just because it doesn't matter. It does matter, because you matter. You and your body are inseparable, and it's time you start loving each other.

You and your body are inseparable, and it's time you start loving each other.

Chapter 2

Let's Get Moving in the Gym

30

When Bethany came to me and said she wanted to add strength training to her exercise routine, I was pleased. Sometimes clients come to me and say they want to lose weight, but they don't want to "bulk up." Many women associate weight training with getting large muscles. Because of the differences in men and women's bodies it is very difficult for most women to obtain a musculature that is as cut and defined as a man's. More importantly, women's physiology doesn't allow them to bulk up the way men do.

Resistance training is very important for women's health, and looking toned and lean are almost secondary benefits. Resistance training strengthens bones and joints. It helps maintain a healthy weight and it stabilizes blood sugar. It helps fight high blood pressure and lower cholesterol.

The basic premise is simple: Ask your muscles to do more than they are used to doing and muscle fibers break down. Afterward, the body rushes in to "heal" the area that has been stressed. The human body doesn't make more muscle fibers; it responds to progressive overload by increasing the size of the fibers that are there. The enhanced muscle fiber has a higher metabolic rate than fat, and so the resting body needs more food than before to maintain itself. As you build more muscle, you enable your body to eat more without gaining weight. If you are following our guidelines for healthy eating, you can further enhance this process and continue to lose fat and gain muscle.

Gaining muscle may indeed cause you to weigh more on your scale, but it will make you leaner. Muscle really does weigh more than fat. Molecularly, fat is not as dense as muscle fiber. As you can imagine, fat is lumpy and deposits unevenly around your body. In most women it tends to collect on the inner thighs, around the waist and hips, on the underside of the arms and the back. Muscle, on the other hand, looks smoother and tighter.

Exercises that do a short number of repetitions at a high weight will make the muscles larger, while exercises that do more repetitions of a lighter weight will elongate the muscles and give them the lean look that women, who are not bodybuilders, want. Imagine the difference between a circus strong man with his 500-pound weight over his head and a wiry long distance runner. Both are quite strong, but the ways the muscles have developed are strikingly different.

If you have tried working out with weights before, you have probably heard many theories about which exercises to do on which days. You may have heard the terminology "Arm Days and Leg Days," or "Upper Body Days and Lower Body Days." In my own life and career as a trainer, I have found that people who work every muscle group during one workout have more overall success with their fitness goals. They tend to retain their new healthy habits. If you are doing resistance training every other day, and you are on an arm/leg schedule, when you miss a day, it can be almost a week before you pay any attention to half your body. Also, where do your all-important core muscles fit into that scenario?

Let's look at eight basic exercises that I started Bethany on. You'll see that each addresses a basic muscle group. If you have experience in the gym, you can start these yourself, and if you don't, you can get a professional at the gym to show you the right way to do the movements so you won't hurt yourself by straining in improper ways. Once you have mastered these exercises, you can use them as your base. With a good knowledge of these muscle groups and movements, as you get stronger and leaner you can modify these eight exercises indefinitely, so that your body continues to be challenged and you continue to be interested. When you are ready to go to the next level, check our website, www.loveyourbodyfitness. com, and you will find a variety of exercises that will work these muscle groups in increasingly challenging and diverse ways.

THE BASIC EIGHT EXERCISES FOR

Chest
Biceps
Shoulders
Legs
Back
Triceps
Lower Back
Abdominals

WHAT IS A WORKOUT?

A warm-up, stretching, strength exercises, cardiovascular exercise, and a quick cooldown/pat on your back for a job well done.

Where can you work out? Anywhere!

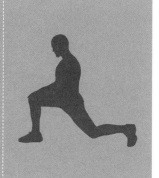

So let's get you warmed up. We'll look at the Basic Eight, the way you'll do them in the gym. In the next chapters, I'll show you how to work these same muscle groups outside, or even at home. Then I'll explain the importance of including cardio in every workout. You're going to love it.

WARMING UP IN THE GYM

DYNAMIC WARM-UP

You don't want to work cold muscles. Always start any workout — cardio or strength — with a warm-up. Gentle movements and stretching will get your circulation going, begin increasing your heart rate, and get some elasticity into your muscles, priming them for their best work, and reducing the risk of injury. Take 5 to 10 minutes to walk briskly, use a step climber or a treadmill, ride a bike, or jog — anything to just get moving. Then stretch from head to toe. Get a systematic stretch routine that gently loosens all your major muscles. While you are stretching, revisit your goals, and get your mind off your day and on your workout. As you stretch, focus on your breathing. Breathe in and out through your nose, concentrating on getting oxygen further down into your lungs. Your breath not only brings good energizing oxygen into your muscles, it also removes waste products. Many of us go around virtually holding our breath, or just using the top part of our lungs. We're not getting a lot of oxygen that way, and it can cause anxiety. During your stretch, get your lungs going, too.

When you stretch, don't do the old static, straight-limb stretches that we all learned in PE, and don't bounce. Gently move your muscles until you can feel them calling out to you and then take a deep breath and move a little further into the stretch. Hold it there for 30 to 60 counts and gently release. Stretching is a good way to check in with your body, and you can do it several times a day — wherever you are. You don't need to save it as a pre-workout routine. If you have back problems or previous injuries, check in with a trainer at your gym and ask for additional stretches to address your needs.

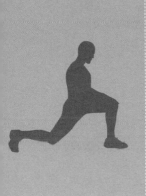

I CANNOT STRESS STRONGLY ENOUGH HOW IMPORTANT WARMING UP AND STRETCHING ARE TO A GOOD WORKOUT. Go for a jog, a brisk walk, a spin on the stairmaster, anything to get your muscles warm and pliable for five, ten, twenty-five minutes, depending on your schedule. Start slowly, feel your body loosen up, and then get your heart rate up. Break a sweat. Don't stop suddenly, but decrease your effort gradually. While you're warming up, pay attention to your breath. Are you taking little sips of air just at the top of your lungs? That's no way to get your system energized. You need to pull that sustaining oxygen deep down into the littlest corners of your lungs. Take deep breaths, and blow them out fully, feeling your lungs fill with air and imagining the oxygen working like a clean fuel throughout your body, powering it up. Once you are warm and pliable, find a spot to stretch.

STRETCHING

I find it easier to stretch systematically so I don't forget a muscle group. Here are the how-tos on some basic stretches. Let's go from the ground up.

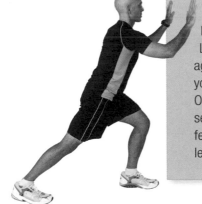

1. Calves
Find a stable object or wall and stand facing it. Lean into the wall at about a 45-degree angle. Push against the wall with your hands and gently push your heels to the ground, or as close as they will go. Once you feel the stretch, hold it there for about thirty seconds to a minute. Breathe into the stretch and feel your muscles letting go. Consciously think about letting them relax.

I find it easier to stretch systematically so I don't forget a muscle group.

2. Quadriceps

Still facing the wall, stand up straight. Use one hand for balance, and reach the other one around behind you. Bend the leg on the same side as the reaching hand at the knee and grab it with your hand at the ankle or foot. Keeping your knee facing down to the ground and being careful not to let your bent leg angle out, bring your bent leg into your glutes until you feel a comfortable stretch. Hold that stretch for thirty seconds to one minute, and repeat on the other side.

3. Hamstrings

Find an elevated surface, and stand facing it about two feet away. Place your foot on it. With your raised knee bent, slowly fold your body over that thigh until your stomach touches your thigh. You should feel a gentle pull in your hamstrings. Keep your back flat like a tabletop from your neck to your tailbone as you hinge down, bending at the hips, not the waist. Hold the stretch where you can feel it, but it is not painful for 30 to 60 counts, and repeat on the other leg. Don't force the hamstrings to go too far too fast, because they can cause you all sorts of woe if you strain them.

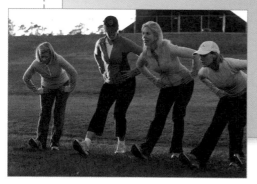

4. Adductors

Spread your legs a little wider than hip distance apart. Lean over so that your elbows are resting on your knees. Gradually shift your weight to one side until you feel the stretch in your inner thighs, hold for 30-60 counts and then move to the other side.

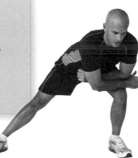

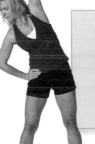

5. Sides and Arms

Stand tall and reach one arm over your head. With both feet firmly on the floor hip distance apart, lean first to one side and then to the other, holding each at the point of tension for 30 seconds to one minute.

35

6. Neck

Slowly look from side to side, up and down, and rotate your head counterclockwise and clockwise, only rotating in a half-circle in the front. Be careful not to force your neck at any point. Using your right hand, reach over your head to your left ear and apply gentle pressure to pull your right ear down towards your right shoulder. Hold the stretch, and repeat on the other side.

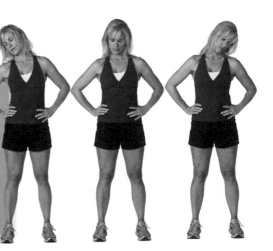

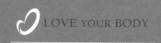

Now, you're stretched and ready. If you came in lethargically, if you had to drag yourself to put your workout clothes on, by this time you should have generated enough energy and endorphins that you are feeling happy and ready to get moving. Take a minute to notice what a brief warm up and stretch can do for your mood.

36

THE BASIC EIGHT:

Just as I believe with a stretch, I find that being systematic in your workout is the best way to feel confident that you are getting everything done in the most efficient way possible. Each exercise will target more than one muscle group, but for simplicity's sake, we will name them for the muscles or area where you'll probably feel the effort the most.

Let's start at the top this time:

1. Chest: Dumbbell Press

Grab a bench and two free weights. It might take a few minutes to determine which size weight you want to use, but take a little time to experiment. You want to be able to do 12-15 repetitions of the same movement. You should feel like the first few repetitions are fairly easy, but the last two or three are quite difficult. You should feel like the last repetition uses the last bit of your strength. Don't worry, because after a short recovery you will feel ready to go again. Sit at the front end of the bench with your legs in front of you and your knees bent about shoulder-width apart. Holding the weights firmly around the middle, place them on your knees and lie back on the bench. Once you are settled, lift the weights on either side of you, even with your chest. Your arms should be out to your sides, bent at the elbow at 90 degrees. Your arms should make one continuous line from elbow to elbow. Keeping the weights parallel to the floor, lift them simultaneously up in a straight line until your arms are straight, but your elbows are not locked. Pause at the top, and slowly, taking as much time to lower them as you took to raise them, lower them to your starting position. Repeat the motion 12-15 times. Remember to breathe out when you are starting to exert yourself on the up push, and inhale as you gradually lower the weights. And keep a good grip on those weights — loving your body means avoiding plastic surgery whenever possible!

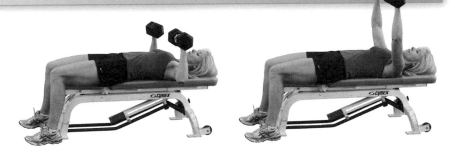

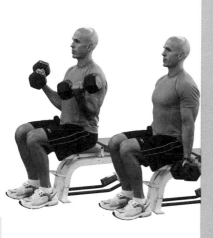

2. Biceps: Bicep Curls

While you're on the bench, you can work your biceps. You'll want two free weights. Sit on the front of the bench, as if you were getting ready to lie down and do chest presses, but don't lie down. Sit up straight and, gripping your weights, hold them on your knees. Looking straight ahead and facing your inner arms straight ahead, lower the weights on each side of you until your arms are straight, but not overextended. Breathing out, bend your arms and lift the weights until they are 45 degrees at the elbows. Your weights will remain parallel to the floor during the entire movement. Once you reach the stopping point on your arc, lower the weights gradually, resisting all the way back to the starting position. The downward trip with weights is just as much a part of the exercise as the lifting phase, and it is important to move smoothly through each phase in a controlled manner. Repeat these movements 12-15 times. If you haven't been doing much exercise at all, you will want to start with two sets, but after four to six weeks, you should be able to do three sets at your proper weight setting. Two to three sets — ladies' choice!

3. Shoulders: Shoulder Press

For your shoulders, you'll want to get two free weights. You can use a flat bench or one that can be angled up like a seat. Sit at the end of the bench with your feet evenly on the floor in front of you, about shoulder-width apart for stability. Bring your weights to shoulder height and hold them so that your palms face away from you. Keeping the angle of each arm even, raise the weights up until your arms are extended over your head. As they move up, the weights should stay in the same plane. Don't let them wobble around side to side, and don't let them come forward or backward. Again, it's easy to remember: 12-15 reps 2-3 times. Getting the hang of it?

4. Legs

Your legs have lots of muscles, so for your introductory exercise set, we're going to work them three specific ways.

4a. Quads: Seated Leg Press

So many people — men and women — seem to respond to this exercise. I'm not sure if it's because we all want our gluteus to be more minimus than maximus, or if it just feels good to sit down for a minute in the gym. Whatever the motivation, this is a great exercise. Find the Leg Press machine in your gym. It's a tilted chair with a big footpad that lifts the weights. There are many variations of this machine, but you'll know it when you see it. Some of them use weights that are added individually to increase the weight, and some of them have all the weights in place and you just move a pin to increase the resistance level. Ask one of the trainers or the gym personnel to help you get set up. Proper use of the equipment and proper form are the best ways to avoid any kind of injury.

Once you're set up on the leg press and have determined your weight level, you'll do your regular routine: 12-15 reps, 2-3 times. You've just gotten to the gym and you already have a routine going. Good work!

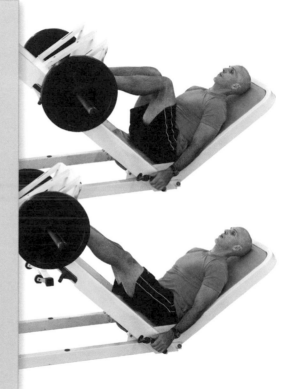

39

Next let's get the hamstrings, those big muscles that run behind your thighs and can cause so much back trouble if they are not strong and stretched.

4b. Hamstrings: Seated Leg Curls

Once you get the machine set for your frame, experiment until you find a good weight setting for your body and fitness level. Sit down on the machine. Make sure your back is against the pad and that your feet are just past the footpad on the end. Secure the leg holder right above your knees and lock into place. Press your heels toward the floor so your knees are at a 90-degree angle and slowly let them up again to the starting position. Always make sure when you are using a machine that the weights settle quietly back onto the stack. Not only is it aggravating to others in the gym to hear the crashing, but also the vibration can break the machine. Repeat the motion 12-15 times for 2-3 sets with a minute break between sets.

40

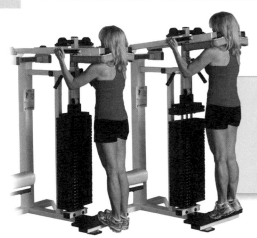

4c. Calves: Standing Heel Raise

Put your shoulders under the pads and place the balls of your feet onto the metal step. Raise your heels as high as you can and then lower them below the normal level of your feet. Repeat the motion as above.

TIP

IF YOU ARE NOT SURE HOW TO GET SET UP ON A MACHINE, DON'T HESITATE TO ASK ANYONE WHO WORKS IN THE GYM OR SOMEONE WHO IS EXERCISING TO HELP YOU FIGURE IT OUT. EVERYONE WAS A BEGINNER ONCE, AND PEOPLE AROUND GYMS TEND TO BE SUPPORTIVE AND ENTHUSIASTIC ABOUT SHARING THEIR INFORMATION.

5. Upper Back: Pull Downs and Back Rows

Your upper back is like your legs — lots of important muscles that contribute to your stability, so we'll work it two ways.

5a. Lat Pull Downs

You can do pull downs on the same machine that you will use for tricep push downs, or you can do them on a machine that is set up exclusively for pull downs. On either machine, you'll want to use the straight bar with the hand grips a little further than shoulder-width apart. Sit facing the weights on the seat, on a big ball, or on a bench. Grip the handles of the bar with your arms extended up and a little to the front. Maintaining a straight spine — as if that string was pulling gently from the top of your head — pull the bar down until it almost touches your chest. As you release it, resist the upward pull, so that your return trip takes as long as your trip down: 12-15 reps, 2-3 sets. Using the ball as your seat will force you to use more of your little muscles in your sides to remain stable, so it can be more challenging. It's a great way to strengthen your core.

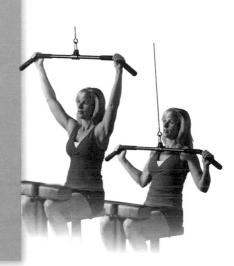

41

5b. Rows (Rhomboids)

For the rows, find a flat bench and a free weight. Put your right hand and your right knee on the bench. With your back as flat as a table, hold the weight in your left hand and let it dangle next to the bench, in front of your straight leg. Keeping the weight in a straight line, lift it up next to your chest so that your arm forms a little triangle or dorsal fin over your back. Hum the theme song to "Jaws" if it makes you feel stronger. Lower your arm slowly, maintaining the resistance. You'll do 12-15 reps on each arm and 2-3 sets, so I think it is easiest to alternate arms — one arm gets a break while the other one is working.

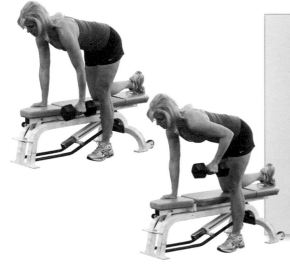

6. Triceps: Push Downs

To work your triceps, those little flying squirrel wings behind your arms, you'll want to find a push down bar. There are all sorts of handles that you can attach to the hook that connects to the cable that lifts the weights, but which one you choose is just a matter of preference — rope, V-bar, straight bar, grips, you'll see a variety sitting on the floor next to the machine. Once your handle is attached, experiment for a minute to determine what weight to set the machine on. As always, you'll want to be able to do 12-15 reps and have to give it some oomph to finish. Once you determine your weight setting, stand facing the stacked weight bars. Grab the handle with both hands, and keeping it level, bring it even with your chest. Stand fairly close to the weights so the cable goes as straight down as possible. Keeping your elbows close to your sides, and keeping them as stationary as possible, push your forearms down until your arms are extended towards the floor. Once you have lifted the weight, resist its drop as you bring your hands back to chest height. Repeat that motion 12-15 times, take a recovery break, and do another set.

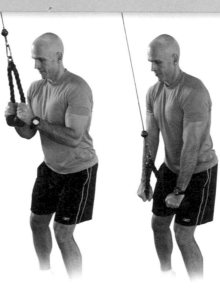

7. Lower Back: 45-Degree Back Extension

This is a fun one, but it might feel a little awkward at first. Think of it as backwards sit-ups. There is a device that looks like something out of a shoeshine parlor. It has a platform for your feet, a padded roll to hold the backs of your ankles in place and a pad for your hips. All aboard! Slide your feet into position, and make sure your hips are high enough up on the pad that you can bend from the hips. Many times I see people placing the pad on their stomachs and bending from the waist. That won't do the trick. Put your upper thighs against the pad, and trust that the feet holders will hold you securely. Now cross your arms like Lily Munster and lower your body towards the floor about 45 degrees. Once you are down, come back up slowly: 12-15 of these will prove quite challenging for most people starting a workout routine, so do as many as you can, and work up to 2 sets. These back extensions are really great for strengthening all the muscles that ache if you spend most of your day sitting.

Now, we're almost done, and I've saved the all-important core for last. Your core muscles are all the muscles in your abdomen and sides that keep your organs in place and steady your limbs. There are many of them, the most frequently mentioned being the abdominals — the stomach muscles that can be called anything from a gut to a six-pack, depending on their condition. All you need to remember is that while everyone wants a flat stomach so they'll look good in clothes, or a bathing suit, or less, the core muscles actually provide us with lots more than good looks — they are the key to a strong body. For your workout in the gym, we'll focus on the abdominals, known as "abs" to their friends.

8. Abs: Knee Lifts

There is a piece of equipment in the gym that looks like an arm chair with no seat. It has a comfortable back and arms, and nothing but air underneath. It is truly the throne of power, because no one sits in it without emerging stronger than when they entered.

Here's how you do it: Climb up and lean your back against the back pad. Place your forearms and elbows on the pads of the seat, and get them comfortable. Firmly grasp the handles and push your tailbone against the back pad. Your weight should now be on your arms. It can be tempting to collapse a little here and sag down, but hold firm and really keep your chest lifted. Now, bend your knees and slowly raise them up until they are even with your stomach — you're sitting in a chair in the air! Try not to grimace when you are doing it, and it will seem easier. Lower your knees slowly, resisting the urge to just drop them like deadweights. Do about 12 -15 repetitions, or as many as you can to start. This is one exercise where your body will let you know — loud and clear — how many reps it can do. Try adding one or two more each time, and challenge yourself to eventually work up to three sets.

44

So you did it! A quick, systematic workout of your whole body.

Now, get that deserved drink of water. You should be hydrating throughout your workout. You can build in little sips or trips to the fountain as your breaks between sets or between exercises. Sweating is your signal that you are working at a level where there is action in your muscles and your body's cleansing system is activated. As you sweat, your body releases toxins. Replacing all that old gunk with lots of clean, fresh water keeps your organs healthy and carries away the by-products of muscle breakdown and manufacture.

Feel good? Those are endorphins at work, and the more regularly you work out, the better you'll feel. In fact, once you make exercise a habit, you'll produce endorphins even when you're not in the gym. And that's a good thing.

If you haven't done any cardiovascular exercise today, now's the time to do it. We'll talk more about the importance of cardio in Chapter Five.

Chapter 3

Getting Outside
with Friends
and Making it Fun

46

An important way to keep your motivation high is to have a workout buddy or a group of buddies. Love Your Body Fitness is all about the positive social experience that creates more energy for everyone involved. Getting outside with a group is a great way to get fresh air, clear your mind, and get fit. Your friends give support when you feel tired, reminding you how much more energy you'll have when you get moving. They can also encourage you to keep working towards that goal when you get frustrated and remind you there is no instant gratification in any worthwhile endeavor. We can fool ourselves with clever rationalizations, but it is much harder to fool our friends! And, aside from all the helpful motivation and support they offer, friendship lightens the load of any work, even a workout. There's nothing like a good laugh to keep you going.

PEOPLE WHO HAVE LOST WEIGHT AND KEPT IT OFF SAY THAT THEIR PRIMARY GOAL WAS TO GET HEALTHY, NOT TO LOSE WEIGHT. Weight loss is a rewarding by-product of lowering your cholesterol and blood pressure and working to feel better and have more energy.

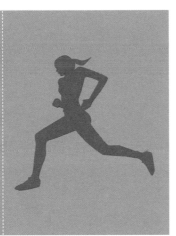

So, lace up those shoes, slather on your sunscreen and find a park or a field near your house. Call a friend or a group on your way out. Take a little bag with you that contains water, a towel, an exercise band, and a medicine ball, 6-12 pounds, depending on your current fitness level.

Just as we did in the gym, I'm going to explain eight basic exercises that you and your friends can do outside. Once you master these, check out our website www.loveyourbodyfitness.com to find the next levels of challenge and a further variety of outdoor exercises to keep you motivated. You'll notice that while you work the same muscles whether you are in the gym or outside,

the exercises I'm describing here tend to address several muscle groups at a time.

As before, let's warm up and stretch. Since you're outdoors now, you've got plenty of room, so I'll explain a dynamic warm-up and stretch.

WARMING UP OUTDOORS

The goal of warming up is to get your circulation going and to loosen your muscles and joints. Always start by standing up straight and pulling oxygen deep into your lungs. Take several deep breaths. As you feel the air enter your lungs, imagine that oxygen carrying energy all through your body. Then blow out the air and the wastes from your body in a strong stream. Reach your arms upward, feeling the pull down your sides, and take a moment to notice the sky — the position of the sun, the cloud cover, the color of the sky. If it's sunny, feel the warmth and energy of the day. If it's cloudy, feel the coolness the cloud cover provides.

Now, get moving. Jog for 5, 10, 25 minutes if you are near a track or a path where you can get some distance, or if you are on a field you can do a series of runners warm-ups. Here are a few that will get you ready to exercise and provide some fun, too.

47

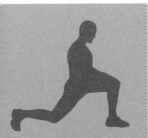

ALWAYS BE IN TOUCH WITH HOW YOU FEEL, WHEN YOU ARE TIRED, WHEN YOU FEEL PAIN. Any workout, whether in the gym, outside, or at home, should first of all be safe and fun. The next factor is variety. I am constantly changing exercises, number of reps, and exercise intensity. Your body will become too efficient if you do the same thing over and over again. Change will cause your body to continue to try to adapt (read that "make more muscle"). That means more strength and cardiovascular endurance. It also means you won't get bored and lose motivation.

High Knees

Find a flat area of grass about 25 yards long. Standing up straight, move across the grassy area at a moderate speed, lifting your knees as high as possible with each stride. Exaggerate the motion so your knees are really high. Stop and take a 30-second breath at the end of the length and then return.

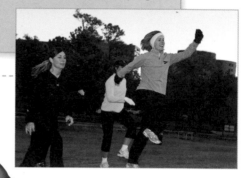

48

Butt Kicks

Stride across the area, and with each stride, touch your heel to your glutes. Move your feet quickly and emphasize the point of contact so it's a staccato motion.

Giant Steps

Just like when you used to play Mother-May-I when you were little, these steps are fun. Step out as far as you can, and really pull hard when you bring the next leg forward. Stay low, and get all those leg and glute muscles working.

Grapevine

Remember those big hulky football players back in high school? Remember watching them do little dance steps across the field and wondering just what they were doing? Called Karaoke or Grapevine, they were working on the dexterity of their feet and also warming up all the muscles on the sides of their legs — abductors and adductors — and also getting into the hip flexors. To do the grapevine, stand sideways and step out with one leg. Cross the second leg past the front of your body. Step out again with the first leg. Now cross the second leg behind your body. Continue to the end of your length this way, alternating stepping in front of your body and behind it. It's much simpler to do than to describe.

Quick Feet

Now take little baby steps, as fast as you can. Get your knees up, but focus most on the speed of your feet. This one may make you laugh out loud!

49

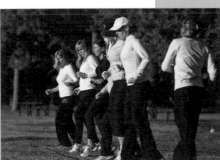

Toy Soldiers

These will warm up your arms as well as your hamstrings. Stand straight up. Step forward with a straight-legged high kick and reach the opposite hand out to touch your toe. Stay straight, tall, and stiff, just like a toy soldier. You'll feel quite warm by the end of your length!

Twists

Imagine doing sit-ups in the air while walking. These are Twists. Put your hands behind your head as if you were doing sit-ups. Bring your knee to your chest and twist, drawing your opposite elbow toward your knee. Step that leg down and out. Bring up the next knee and twist to the other side. Continue down your length. You'll definitely feel this in your sides.

Animal Walks

There is no end to the imaginative animal walks you can do, and each will warm up and stretch various parts of your body. Bear Walking, with your legs straight and your hands on the ground will stretch out your hamstrings and your glutes. Crab Walking, with your hands behind you and your knees bent up will warm up and stretch your quads and your arms. Inchworms, where you start by standing, bend your knees, touch the ground and walk forward with your hands until you are in a push up position, and then walk your feet up to your hands and start over. This will warm up your whole body!

After several minutes of lengths, you'll be in high spirits and ready to work hard. Take a moment to mentally run through your body, checking from head to toe to see if any stiffness remains or if you have not warmed up any little muscles. Reach up to the sky again and take a few deep breaths. Ready to go?

51

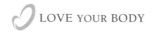
THE GREAT OUTDOORS BASIC EIGHT

1. Chest: Push-Ups

We skipped push-ups when we got started in the gym, but we can never leave this fabulous exercise by the wayside for too long. The push-up is one of the great exercises of all time. You'll notice when you go through this outdoor routine that most of these exercises are designed to target more than one muscle at a time. When you do your push-ups, notice how not only are you feeling it in your arms, but that your chest and your shoulders are invited to the party, too.

Let's talk form first. Get on your knees — I could say "Drop and give me twenty" here, but I'll refrain — and place your hand shoulder-width apart in front of you on the ground. Here you have a choice. There are two ways to do basic push-ups. For beginners, you will keep your knees on the ground as you lower your nose close to the ground between your hands. For standard push-ups, you will raise your knees off the ground, so that your back forms a tabletop. I recommend starting with your knees on the ground until you build up considerable strength in your muscles. It is just too tempting to arch your back or sag like an old donkey if you are not quite strong enough to do the standard style push-up. But don't worry. One of the great things about push-ups is that it is remarkable how much improvement you will see in just a little time. Before long, you'll be up on your toes giving me 20, 30 and more push-ups. So just start slowly and get your form down.

Whatever your push-up style, try to do just one more after you think you want to quit. That will be the number you want to beat the next time.

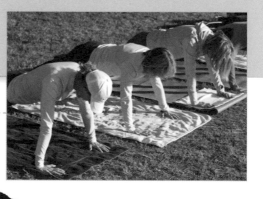

2. Biceps: Band Curls

While we're outside, we'll work your biceps with bands, which are available at any store that carries fitness equipment, and they come in several resistances. They are like tubular rubber bands with handles, and you can use them for many different exercises. We particularly like them because you can take them with you when you travel.

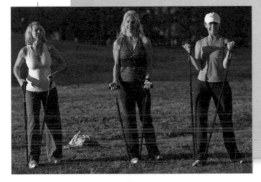

To use the bands for your biceps, stand in the middle of the band with one or both feet depending on how difficult it is for you. Using just one foot will provide a little less resistance. Keeping your upper arms firm, bend your elbows and bring your hands up to your shoulders. Resist the band as you straighten out your arms. Repeat 12-15 times, for 2-3 sets. Does this sound familiar?

53

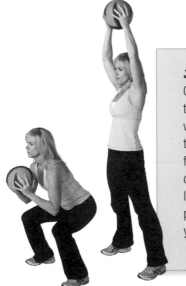

3. Shoulders: Squat with Medicine Ball Shoulder Press

Grab a medicine ball and hold it chest-level with your elbows pointing towards the ground at about a 45-degree angle. Place your feet shoulder-width apart with your toes pointing out slightly like a penguin. Think of your back as a flat tabletop that cannot curl up or arch. Sit on an imaginary chair, until your legs form a 90-degree angle, and keep your knees over your toes. Feel tippy? That's ok. Here's the really fun part: After you sit in your imaginary chair, stand up and lift your medicine ball up over your head. You've gotten a squat and a shoulder press all in one package. It's a great combination, and to keep your balance, you're engaging lots of great core muscles.

4. Legs: Lunges

I can hear you groaning already, but stay open-minded here. The lunge is your friend. It is one of the easiest, most versatile and most portable exercises ever invented. In fact, up there with the push-up, it could almost be considered an "all-you-ever-need" exercise. But we all need a little variety.

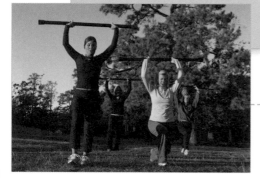

54

With all exercises — whether with free weights, machines or plyometrics (bodybuilding, jump training) — using good form is the key to maximizing and targeting the benefit and avoiding injury. Good form for the lunge means a straight spine, supported by tight abs. It means moving smoothly and slowly through the motion, not jerking to get it over with. It means a gradual transfer of your weight. Once you start doing add ons (with medicine balls, free weights, hops, whatever you like) your basic good form will become even more important.

Stand at the end of an open area, long enough to take about 25 big steps. Face forward with your legs together. Step out comfortably with your right leg until your legs are between 45 and 90 degrees apart. Drop your back knee — the left one — until it is about 6 inches off the ground. Using the force in your right glute, push forward, stepping out on your left leg. Do 20-25 of these lunges, depending

LUNGES ENGAGE YOUR HAMSTRINGS AS THE SECONDARY MUSCLE GROUP. You work your hamstrings when you do butt kicks. When you are outside, you are constantly engaging your leg muscles!

on your space and energy. It's a simple, natural movement.

Make sure that you come down smoothly and deeply on your back leg, and make sure that you are using your glute force rather than your quadriceps to make the step forward. Many of your leg muscles will feel the lunge, but you can choose which muscle will carry the bulk of the load.

Modify your steps so that you are balanced and not teetering. You'll use the lateral muscles, the ones down your sides, for support, and that's another big benefit of the lunge. While you are getting the hang of lunging, you can hold your arms out for balance. Later, your own legs will keep you balanced, and you can use your arms to add weight or nuance to the exercise.

Do 2-3 sets of lunges, depending on your fitness level. At first, you will think that your legs and bottom are burning up and that you won't be able to take another step, but you will find that your body recovers quickly. Don't save your strength for the next set. That burn is your proof that you're loving your body in the most passionate way possible. Think of that feeling as burning love, and get after it!

5. Back

We'll use the bands for these exercises, and you'll need to find a tree or a pole. You can share it with a friend or two. If you are outside on a hot day, it will probably feel a little cool and shady under your tree, and that's an added benefit.

5a. Band Lat Pulls

Wrap the band around your tree or a pole one time and make sure it is stable. Face your tree, bend your knees slightly and bend forward at the hips until your back is parallel to the floor. Pull the handles of the bands back toward your body in a slow, even motion, and resist on the way back. Do 12-15 reps, 2-3 sets, depending on your fitness level.

If your friends can do lots more reps than you can, don't let it drive you up the tree, just do one more rep than you did last time and keep smiling — that's how you love your body. One of our important beliefs at Love Your Body is that other people, trainers included, are there for companionship and encouragement, not to yell at you, to shame you, or to compete with you. If we wanted you to be comparing your Lat Pulls with everybody else's, we'd call our boot camps Love Everybody Else's Body and Try to Make Yours Keep Up. Your body, your lat pulls, your reps and your sets. Love it!

5b. Band Rows

Just like you used the pull down machine in the gym to work your back, you'll use your band outside. Go back to your tree. Wrap your band around it, and face it. With your knees slightly bent, pull the handles of the band toward you until your elbows are behind your body. Smooth motions, row, row, row your boat, 12-15 times, 2-3 sets. What a routine!

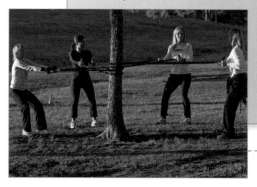

6. Triceps: Dips

This is a fun exercise to do outside. Find a bench, a short wall, or even a ledge at the park. Face away from the bench and squat down. Raise your elbows behind you, and place the palms of your hands on the bench with your fingers pointing forward. Your hands will bend at the wrists at a 90-degree angle. Scoot your feet out in front of you and keep your knees bent. You should look like a tippy tabletop. Slowly bend your elbows and lower your body, keeping your back fairly straight. Once your elbows are completely bent, slowly straighten them, lifting yourself up without locking your elbows. Try to do 12-15 dips, 2-3 times. Feel some core muscles kicking in?

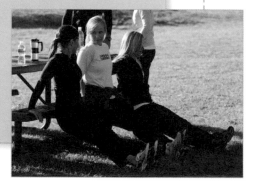

7. Lower back: Superwoman

Superwoman. The name says it all. This is one of our favorite exercises in the Love Your Body Boot Camps, and with all the variations that are possible I hope it will become one of your favorites, too. Here are the basics: You extend your arms and legs and you fly. Since gravity will no doubt keep you from actual lift off, you'll need to use a little imagination here. Lie flat on your stomach. Extend both arms in front of you. Now lift your legs, press your pubic bone into the ground, and reach in front of you as hard as you can. Feel the breeze underneath you? If that doesn't do it for you, you can use right leg, left arm and then left arm right leg. Or, you can get on all fours and lift the opposing limbs. In this case, a picture says a thousand words, so take a look at the possibilities, and just know that 12-15 repetitions of any of these superwoman exercises, executed in 2-3 sets will leave you feeling like Lynda Carter all under.

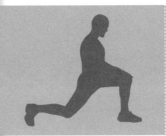

IN THE AT-HOME EXERCISE SECTION, I'LL SHOW YOU HOW TO DO SUPERWOMAN WITH THE LEGS LIFTED.

57

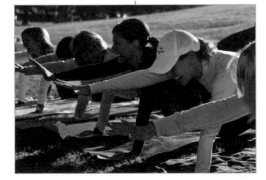

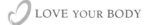

8. Abdominals: The Plank

Feeling like a Superhero? We've already worked your other seven key body parts, let's go right for the core. Get a towel and get ready for that burning love!

The plank has many names, and you will find it in many diverse exercise systems — yoga, martial arts, bodybuilding, pylometrics, and more — and no matter what you call it, when you mention it to anyone who has worked out for any time, you will get a knowing, respectful look. Plank, burning bridge, bridge of fire, top of the push-up, you get the picture.

Here's how you do a basic plank: Lie on your stomach on your towel and bring your arms to chest/shoulder level, wherever you would be comfortable doing a push-up. Now, keeping your forearms on the ground, palms down, push up so your body forms a table. Make sure your back is straight and your bottom is not poking up in the air. Your lower back is strong. Just stay there. Simple. You will soon notice the burning sensation in your stomach, and you'll desperately want to drop down. Don't do it. Hold the plank as many counts as you can without collapsing.

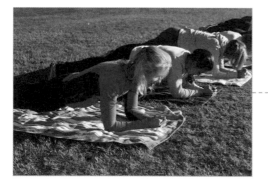

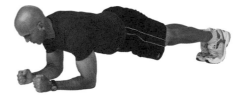

The plank is a real winner, and it will make you feel like one, too — after you get through the part where it makes you feel like yelling

Set a goal for yourself. Can you plank for only 20 seconds the first time? That's ok. Rest a minute and then try to do 20 seconds again. Do three planks. The next time you workout, try to go 10 seconds longer. Although planking feels intense while you are doing it, it is remarkable how quickly you'll build up your endurance, and how good you'll feel when you reach a minute, two minutes, and even five! Here's another twist — the Side Plank. Lie on your side. Stack your feet, one on top of the other, parallel to the floor. Keeping your legs straight and firm, push up with your lower hand, so that your arm is extended. Your sides should be facing the sky and the ground. Reach your top arm slowly over your head and push your top side up towards the sky. If you can, drop your head back and look at the clouds. Feel both sides working — your top side stretching and your lower side contracting. Hold your side plank for a number of counts — can you do 30, or 60?

Then drop down slowly. Repeat on the other side, recover and then do both sides again. If you are feeling strong, do one more set. You can also do the straight arm plank.

As you increase your times, you will see direct results in your abs and your sense of inner strength. The plank is a real winner, and it will make you feel like one, too — after you get through the part where it makes you feel like yelling. And if you want to yell, that's ok, too. Our promise is just that we won't yell at you!

After that last plank, roll over onto your back and gaze up at the sky. Take a deep breath and feel the blood coursing through your muscles. Ready for that cardio? At our boot camps, one of our favorite outdoor cardio exercises is Horses. Check out Chapter Five and I'll give you some general cardio pointers to get you pedalling/running/hopping in the right direction.

59

Chapter 4
Home Alone

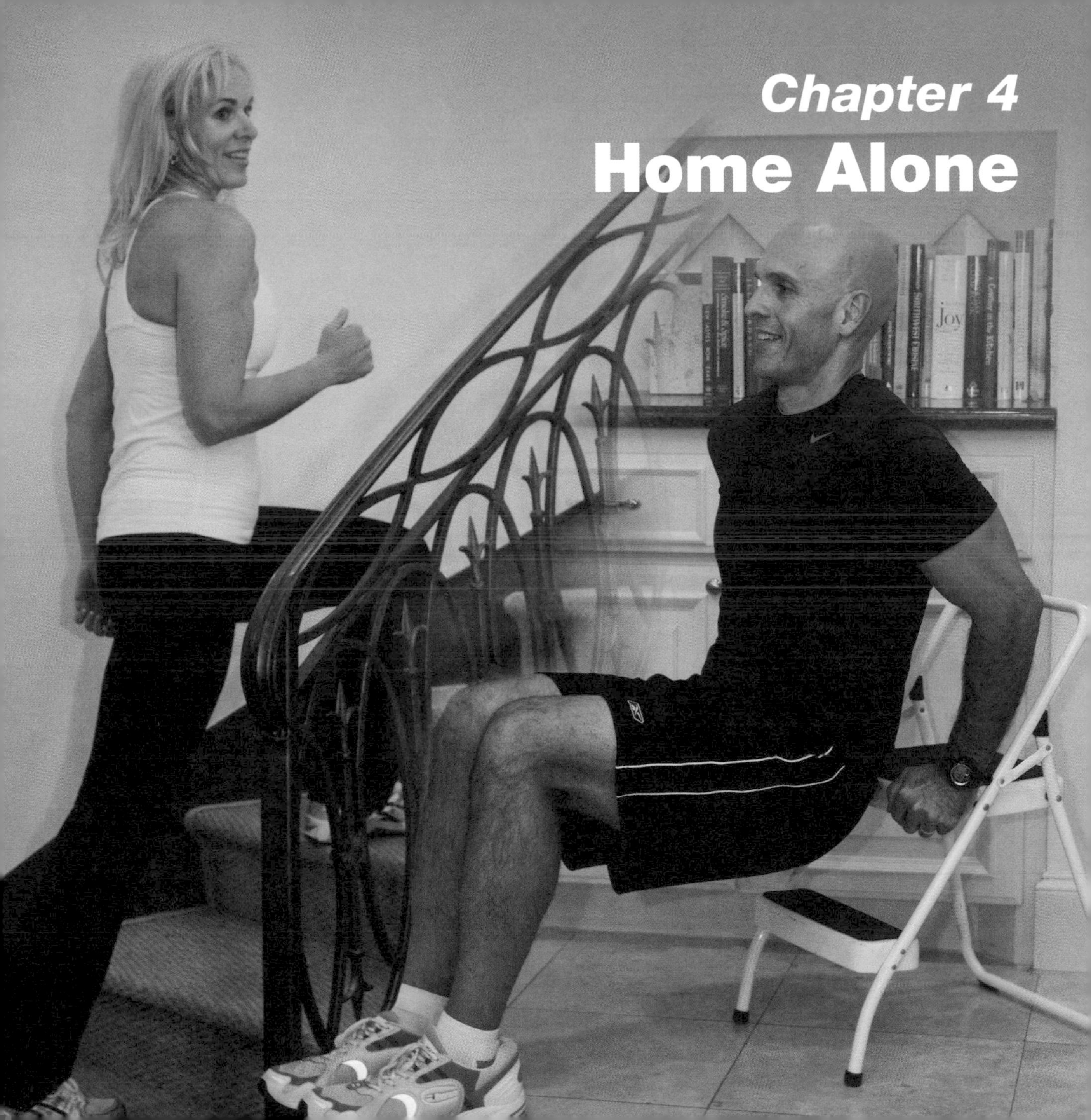

So your buddies are all out at the gym or at work, and you're stuck at home with (choose one) the new baby, the sick child, the broken appliance and the repairman's vague schedule. Guess you'll just have to wait until tomorrow to get that strength workout in, right? Wrong, wrong, wrong. I'm not yelling here, I just want you to know how strongly I feel that this is the place where so many women get off the fitness highway. They exit when little complications like this come up, and they just put down roots at the rest stop. A change in schedule at home or a family vacation or a business trip that might keep you inside doesn't need to prevent you from loving your body.

And it's important to look at it that way: Taking the 30 to 45 minutes that you will need to take care of yourself properly isn't selfish; it's actually the best thing to do for everyone involved. It is so much easier to love everybody else when you love yourself.

You've probably noticed the pattern that I've been setting up. I want you to do a series of eight exercises that address every major muscle group in your body: 15 repetitions of each exercise and 2-3 sets of repetitions. Between sets you should take a break for recovery and hydration. See? I told you you'd be your own trainer in no time.

The key to getting your workout at home is to do the same thing you'd do in the gym or outside with your friends. Your space and equipment will be different, but add a little imagination, and you'll get the same results.

A change in schedule at home or a family vacation or a business trip that might keep you inside doesn't need to prevent you from loving your body.

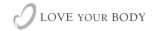

BASIC EIGHT AT HOME

1. Chest: Push-Ups or Chest Press

Push-ups outside were fun; how about 2-3 sets on the floor now? You'll feel it in your chest as well as the shoulders and arms. If you aren't interested in more push-ups now, grab something that weighs about 10 pounds (how about that adorable three-month-old baby?), lie down on your back, and hold it over your chest with both hands and lift it —15 reps, 2-3 sets. If you do choose to do chest presses with your baby, do them very slowly and gently and never shake the baby. And please, just as you do with weights in the gym, put the baby back in the proper place with care.

The important thing to remember is that people used to stay fit before anyone invented the dumbbell. Back when fields had to be plowed and clothes were washed by hand, the business of life was good exercise. You've heard that many times, but the trick now is to tell yourself that it doesn't matter what you're lifting, it matters that you are systematically moving your muscle groups against resistance.

Now, you get the picture. You'll move through the groups, doing the motions I taught you in our gym workout section, but substituting an object you have at home. You'll notice that push-ups and planks don't change whether you are inside or out. I used to like thinking about the Count of Monte Cristo — keeping his mind and his body fit in just a small cell. As long as you have space enough to do a push-up, you can keep yourself fit.

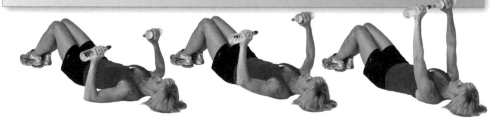

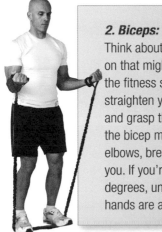

2. Biceps: Curls

Think about water bottles, moonstones from your garden, anything you can get a grip on that might weigh about 8-10 pounds, or get an elastic cord with handles from the fitness store. Easily transportable, you can take it wherever you go. Stand or sit, straighten your back, and extend your arms down. If you are using a band, step on it and grasp the handles. If you are holding objects, hold tight. Most people forget that the bicep muscle goes past your elbow, so get the full extension. As you bend those elbows, breathe out, keeping them near your sides and lifting your hands in front of you. If you're using a band, you'll feel strong resistance. Move your arms about 90 degrees, until your palms face your chest. As you slowly release, breathe out until your hands are at the starting position: 15 reps, 2-3 sets. You know the drill.

65

3. Shoulders: Lateral-Shoulder Raise with something handy

Don't have a bench at home? Not many of us do. But everybody has a stool or a chair. If you have free weights at home, great. If you don't, or you're on the road, find something with a little heft to it. A gallon water jug with a handle? That'll work. A little bronze statue? A big dictionary? Be creative. Take that object, and hold it carefully out to the side. With your elbows slightly bent, raise your arms laterally. Depending on what you choose, you might need to do more than 15 reps to feel the burn in your shoulders. Maybe try 20 or 25. Keep trying, and if you wish, invest in a couple of hand weights. I like the concept of using what you have, but do what is easiest for you! Stop and recover when you feel the muscles working but before they are straining. Or, for a variation on shoulder raises, get that band out and stand on it, placing it under your feet. Hold the handles in each hand and raise them up, mimicking a cheerleading move you used back in the day. Resist up and down: 15, 2-3. Go Team!

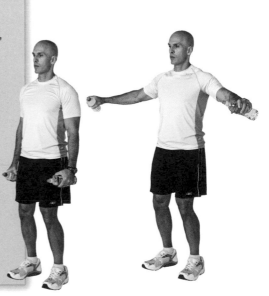

4. Legs: Stairway to Heaven

Are you old enough to remember when every school dance ended with "Stairway to Heaven" so everybody would have one last chance to hug on the one they loved? It's like that here, except the one you're loving is you! Consider the stairs as your slow dance with yourself. You'll definitely get all hot and bothered, but you'll feel so good when you're done. The great thing is, you'll respect yourself even more! Take a deep breath of that good oxygen-filled air surrounding you and head for the stairs. Now up you go. Break it up. Go up the first time running as fast as you can. Lope down, and go up again, taking them two at a time. Go up again, stretching to three at a time. You're slowing down, but you're still using lots of power. How do you feel? Three sets of three might be enough for you at this point. Or, if you still have energy to burn, do another set, first taking three steps at a time, then two, then one. Leave it all on the dance floor — there's nothing to save it for after this — the party's over until next time. Do step-ups on your front stoop! Step up and down — pretend you are in an aerobic class from the 80s!

Just remember that it's supposed to be fun. Don't overexert yourself, or you'll just try to get out of it next time. I can't stress enough that the keys to maintaining interest and commitment to an exercise program are variety, increasing your intensity as you improve, and fun — and the fun can be had anywhere you are, with old friends, new friends, or even by yourself.

Just warming up? Feeling good? Lunge around that house. Pick up some dirty dishes or some of your kids' clothes off the floor as you go. Or dust. There are lots of ways to take your mind off your pain when you lunge around the house. Just keep your form. Stand straight, move up and down in slow, steady movements, and lower your back knee almost to the floor.

5. Back

Have we been ignoring your lats? Not as much as you might be worrying because they have been at work during your lunges and push-ups, engaging to help you keep that balance. But let's give them some good attention of their own now. If you have resistance bands, they usually come with a door clamp. Read the instructions well to clamp it on and then go for it.

5a. Lat Pulls

Bend 30 degrees and grab both handles. Pull parallel to your body and repeat. Just like we did outside, but this time the beautiful flowering pear tree is your laundry room door. Imagination helps a lot in an indoor workout.

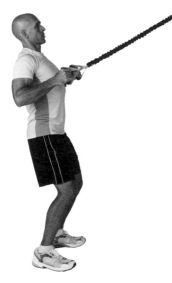

5b. Rhomboids: Rows

Stay upright and pull the handles perpendicular to your body on this one: 12-15 reps, 2-3 sets, some things don't change, no matter where you are.

If you don't have a resistance band, try pulling your garden hose off the hose roller to get your lats working, or pull laundry out of the dryer (that might get dull 12-15 times in a row). Anything that you need to pull toward your body that offers some resistance. For your rhomboids, you can do rows on your coffee table, or you can bend at the hips and support yourself with your straight arm on your big cylinder kitchen trashcan while you lift your 10-pound objects.

6. Triceps

To work your triceps, you have lots of options. You can find a bench or a step and dip, just as we did outside in the park. You can also do wall push-ups. Stand facing the wall and lift your hands, palms against the wall, just over shoulder level. Keeping that body straight, lean into the wall with your elbows close to your sides. Now push yourself back. Feel those triceps working? Try to do 2-3 sets of 15, resisting as you come towards the wall and as you push away from it. You'll get the added benefit here of engaging other muscles as well as your triceps.

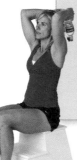

Another easy way to work your triceps at home is to grab a bottle of bleach or a heavy water bottle and put it behind your head. Hold on with both hands and point your elbows to the ceiling at a 45-degree angle. Extend your arms until the hands are straight above your head without locking your elbows. Slowly lower both hands down behind your head: 12-15 reps, 2-3 sets.

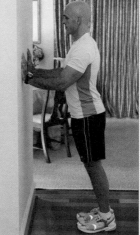

7. Lower Back: Superwoman on Hands and Knees

Here is your chance to be a Super Hero again. Get on all fours. If you have dogs, put them in another room, because they will think you want to play and come over and lick you in the face. It is a little distracting. Once you are on all fours, make your back table-flat. Raise one arm and the opposite leg and extend them. Hold them out for a set number of counts. You'll know what the right number is — you'll feel the muscle engage, but not feel a strain. Then repeat the motion with the other arm and leg. Try to do 12-14 reps, 2-3 times.

As with any back exercise, really listen to your body. You can't love anyone you don't communicate with. When your back says, "We are moving from healthy tension into stress," stop. Don't ever move into pain. Whoever invented the "no pain, no gain" school of exercise must have had stock in heating pads and aspirin, but they did not have your most successful healthy lifestyle in mind. Do your Superwoman carefully, at your own pace, and your back will thank you every time you bend down and pick something up!

69

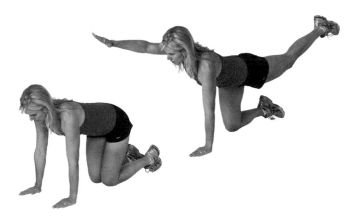

8. Abdominals: Hip lifts

Hip lifts are just like backwards sit-ups. It seems like lots of exercises are like reverse sit-ups. Tastes like chicken. But the point is, sit-ups activate your core — and so do these exercises, just in different ways, focusing on different muscles. Here's what you'll do for a hip lift:

Lay flat on the ground. Raise your legs into the air and point your feet to the ceiling. Gently lift your hips off the ground and lower them back down. The movement is basic here, but the form is important. Your legs might try to swing out to the side – don't let them. Keep your movements small, and don't use momentum to lift your legs back up. You are in control of this exercise, not your legs. After you've done 12-15 of these babies (test yourself, because you might be able to do 20, as long as you are not overdoing it), 2-3 times, you are done with your fabulous at-home workout. Who says you need a gym to be fit?

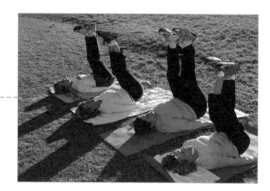

Love Your Heart – Cardio Is King

IT'S CARDIO TIME

Now you've worked the Basic Eight, inside, outside, or at home. You're feeling good, and it's time for Cardio. Cardiovascular exercise, just another way to say we all need to move our bodies every day. Aim for every day as your goal, or if you are just starting to get fit, try for every other day at first. You say, "I don't have enough time," but your body can't tell time. All it knows is it was built for movement.

72

Cardiovascular exercise, just another way to say we all need to move our bodies every day.

If you can walk two times a day for 15 minutes (as briskly as possible) that is all your heart needs to be on the healthy track. But to really feel good and be lean, you need to bump that up and continue to push yourself. Could you just jog to the end of the block? Could you add a sprint or a run? Moving your body will make you feel like a kid again — I promise!

The more you do, the better you feel. There are all types of cardio exercises you can do: In the gym, there is a variety of wonderful machines. Outside you can run sideways, karaoke/grapevine around a track, skip, bunny hop, just change it up. You will get stares, but if you are doing these things with other friends, you'll all be giggling. And, oh, yes, while you have your buddies, don't forget to bear crawl. Or do mountain climbers, or squat thrusts…the list is endless. If there are stairs at your house, use them. And there is always jogging.

I promised to share one of our favorite cardio exercises. Horses (or what we heard called less favorably "Suicides" in our '70s gym classes) are a great way to end a workout. They'll leave you with lots of endorphins and the feeling that you have really worked hard. So let's get up off the floor, or the grass, or the rug, and take that warm body for a little run.

Find an open area and set up three markers — 10 yards, 20 yards and 30 yards away from the start. Ready? Set? Now sprint to the first marker, bend down, touch it and sprint back as fast as you can. Touch the start, sprint to the second marker and sprint back. Touch the start, sprint to the last marker, touch it, and run as fast as your little legs can carry you back to the start. Was that hard? It was supposed to be. Walk around, breathing deeply, take a sip of water, and recover. You should take about as much time to recover as it took you to do that first horse. In the beginning, don't get frustrated with yourself if it takes a little longer to step up to the start again, or if you find that you have to jog in the last leg. Stick with it a few sessions, and you'll see improvement in less time than you'd imagine.

The eventual goal will be to do three sets, as fast as you can go. Remember — push yourself a little further each time. As it gets easier, add additional cones so that each horse has four or even five legs. You'll know when you are ready. You know your body — now love it!

When you are done, whether it is the first time or the 50th, your heart will be pounding, and you will be sweaty. You should feel great and energized but not feel dizzy or clammy. Pacing yourself, and pushing yourself at a

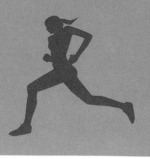

comfortable rate is one of the keys to getting and staying in shape. If you try to get in shape in one day, at best you will dread coming out the next time and at worst you will hurt yourself. Working out should be challenging, yet fun. Remember, friends who join you to work out are there to inspire and support you, not to compete with you. You win merely by being out there and moving that body.

Let's look further into this fitness magic called cardio with some help from Vince.

Before I go further into cardiovascular exercise, let me say something about perceived exertion (PE). Let's use a 1-10 scale. Level one is at rest and 10 means you can't exercise any harder or maximum exertion. With a new client, I start them out at a 6. I like this scale better than heart rate, because YOU have to be the judge of where to start. Another good rule of thumb is you have to be able to carry on a conversation during the cardiovascular exercise. I have some clients who push themselves and are motivated to get to a point where they can talk, but their PE is an 8 or a 9.

Clients ask me all the time: What is the best exercise cardio equipment? That's an easy answer: Whatever you will use! Remember, it's not the equipment that makes a difference, it is moving your body. Eat less, move your body more. No secrets between us! I do think it's important to mix it up. First, and most importantly, your body responds well to change. Second, boredom is the kiss of death to any workout routine. So use different cardio equipment regularly. Change it up all the time. Change the intensity. Keep your body guessing. Never let it know what is around the next corner. Never let it get into a routine that says, "Every Monday is bike! Tuesday is a run!" Shock your body. You can do a long slow burn (PE of about 6) one day and interval training the next day. Or, use three different machines in one day with slow burn. Then the next day try interval training on one machine. Just keep moving. Keep those endorphins flowing.

Many people will get on a bike for 30 minutes on the same level every workout. They're definitely burning calories, but varying equipment and resistance can make bigger changes in your body. Bethany is an example of this trend. When she came to me, she was a single machine/single intensity exerciser. She noticed huge differences after she began mixing up her cardio workouts. Here are some of the different machines I recommended to her and some pointers about using each one.

Treadmill:

Most people get on the treadmill and walk at a steady pace or even run at a set speed. Bethany was a runner and had not walked on a treadmill in years. I challenged her to walk at 3.0 on a level 12% grade. She was shocked at the sweat she broke and the workout she got. She was amazed at how quickly she became tired. Over time she has changed her body and has increased her incline to 15% grade and even 30% grade. On the treadmill, the important thing is not to hold on the machine with a death grip, but to slow your speed enough so you don't need the machine for support.

Stationary Bike:

A steady pace on the stationary bike is fine, but try changing the resistance. Even try standing up in the saddle and at the same time changing resistance on the bike. Vary your resistance, starting at 30-second intervals. Gradually work your way up in time. The important thing is to push yourself enough so that you enjoy it, but you are still challenging yourself. Only you can motivate yourself, and only you will know if you actually got "a good workout."

Elliptical:

Most elliptical machines have incline and resistance settings. I suggest changing both frequently and pedaling forward and backwards. Use the RPMs as your guide and interval train at PEs of 5 to 8.

Stair climber:

Many stair climbers have program settings. Try using the interval or speed-interval setting for a killer workout. You can set the level, and then change it any time if it wears you out. Don't worry, just keep stepping!

Other Cardio Machines:

Most gyms will also have other cardio machines. Make it a point to try them and have someone teach you how to use them. Remember jogging, walking briskly, swimming, biking, jumping rope with your little girl, anything that gets and keeps you moving at a rate that increases your heart rate is wonderful. Don't get too bogged down in heart rate monitors and equipment. The more moving parts involved in your workout means the more parts that can break. Can't you hear that rationalization: "I can't get any cardio in today…I can't find my heart-rate monitor." Love may mean never having to say you're sorry, but loving your body means never making excuses. If it's raining, hit those stairs. Run around the house. You've got to move it, move it! (Note singing lemurs in the background!)

So, there you have it. This is the program that has been successful for my clients in the gym and at boot camp. This is what I have Bethany do, and it has worked wonders for her.

75

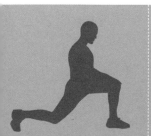

I KNOW THAT THERE WERE TIMES, ESPECIALLY IN THE BEGINNING, THAT BETHANY THOUGHT I WAS MERCILESS, BUT SHE CAN TELL YOU MORE ABOUT THAT. ALL I KNOW IS what I see, and what I see is a very fit lady.

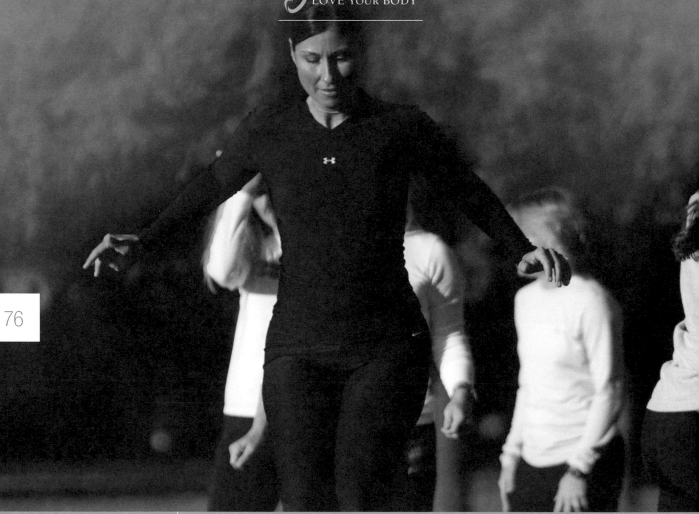

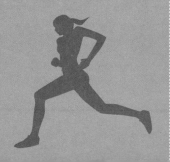

WELL, VINCE IS RIGHT. He was merciless sometimes, but I'm glad he made me stick with it. His strength-training system is the only program that I have been able to continue on my own without a trainer actually taking me through it. After I learned the basics, I found that I had enough strength to motivate myself to improve, and when I plateaued I would go back to Vince and get the next level of repetitions, or some new exercises for the same muscle groups to add variety. As you've probably figured out, variety is important to me.

NO CHOICE

First of all, don't even give yourself a choice not to exercise. If you're tired, if you're sad, if you're busy, no matter what — unless you are physically ill — tell yourself that you will exercise. "This is what I do." If you are sick, tell yourself not to exercise, because your body needs to work on healing, not to work on building muscles. But if you are well, no excuses. Don't sacrifice your workout time to do one more thing for your husband or your children, or your job. Don't try to check a few e-mails. Put your exercise first, and you will have more energy for the people and the demands in your life. This is critical. Many people say they don't have time to exercise. When you start exercising, you suddenly find you have more time, because you have more energy. Respecting and valuing my exercise time was one of the hardest things for me to accomplish before it became a habit. I was always thinking something else was more important. Luckily, I had Vince there, and he took no excuses. If you think you are going to try to write yourself a note to get out of gym class, get a group of buddies to work out with. They can remind you that you are at least as important as everybody else, and you'll be doing everybody else a favor by being fitter, happier and healthier. You need someone who is counting on you to be there until you can trust yourself to do it alone. It helps if your workout partners can make you laugh, too.

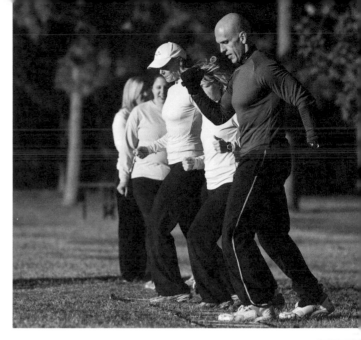

Another realization about working out regularly is that I had to be honest with myself. It was easy to say that's all I can do, but when I realized that I really wanted to get fit, doing less than I possibly could was cheating myself, taking away an opportunity to get as fit as possible. You know when you can do more. Sweat, sweat, sweat: If you don't, you're not working hard enough. The rule I set for myself is: If I can wear my exercise clothes the next day, I haven't worked hard enough. If they are wet and gross, toss them in the hamper and feel great about that workout. If you really don't like to sweat, just remind yourself that it washes right off.

Don't sacrifice your workout time to do one more thing for your husband or your children, or your job.

Chapter 6
Choose Your Food – Why We Hate Diets

WE'RE NOT NUTRITIONISTS, BUT WE KNOW WHAT WORKS...AND WHAT DOESN'T!

Organic, locally grown, vegetarian, lacto-vegetarian, low-fat, low-carb, grapefruit, cabbage soup, protein shakes, hardboiled egg, you name it. From North Beach to South Beach, you can find many diets that friends will swear have helped them to lose five, ten, twenty or more pounds. We tried many of them ourselves. We have friends who are nutritionists, and we have been given lots of specific diets to follow that do indeed help us to drop those pounds. But dropping pounds and being fit are two different things. Unfortunately, some pounds, which we've lost on a diet, have come right back. The pounds we lost on the cabbage soup diet stayed off until we got sick of eating cabbage soup. Then we tried hardboiled eggs. The story is the same. Diets just don't work for very long.

WHEN REACHING YOUR GOAL — AND YOU WILL — NEVER JUST QUIT. It is important to see exercise and healthy eating as a lifestyle, a commitment for the rest of your life. I have a number (a round one) that is my stop number. When I wake up close to 140 pounds, I get right back on the horse and really focus on my nutrition! I kick it up a notch, so to speak. Numbers aren't important in how we define ourselves, but they can act as an objective guide once we discover where we ought to be to feel our best.

Remember to embrace those who help you. So many people say, "How can I diet when my assistant brings us all hamburgers and fries?" Tell the assistant when you say you want a hamburger, that really means, 'Bring me a grilled chicken salad!'" Watch restaurant portion sizes. My mom still shudders at the current "SUPER-sized meals." She says that in the '50s and '60s, portions were so much smaller. Remember you can have a "to go" box brought when your meal comes. Take half out and save it.

Listen to your body when it tries to tell you that you're full. This may be the first time you've ever really listened to it. It takes about 20 minutes after you eat before you feel full. Eat slowly and wait before you continue serving yourself another helping of mashed potatoes!

We are all too familiar with the yo-yo effect that occurs when we lose weight and then, within weeks or months, gain it all back. Nothing is more discouraging — all that hard work for nothing! Scientists have explained this effect by showing us how hunger and body fat are regulated through an appetite control center in the hypothalamus, a part of the brain that regulates many body functions. We each have our own hypothalamic "set point," often determined by genes and usually very resistant to change. This setting is designed to keep us at a certain weight and is the main reason that dieting is so frustrating. As we reduce our food consumption and caloric intake, the hypothalamus signals our metabolism to compensate by more efficiently storing fat. When we go off the diet, our bodies will gain back the weight we lost. In long-term diets, our bodies will plateau. The less we eat, the less weight we seem to be losing.

Plus, who eats every meal at home these days? It's impossible to find a restaurant that offers every dish on a strict-diet plan and a scale for measuring portions.

What we need is not a diet, but a master plan: A way of eating that can be adapted to our specific lifestyles and all the unforeseen complications that arise every day. We need a food plan that enhances our exercise routine. It sounds too good to be true, but it's not. We'll give you the basics, and show you how to have it your way, as the old Burger King ad used to promise.

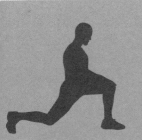

I THINK MANY OF US USE GENETICS AS AN EXCUSE FOR BEING OVERWEIGHT. In reality, our behavior is to blame. Sucking down a double cheeseburger, fries and four beers can't be blamed on our parents. We have to realize that we're simply eating too much and that restaurant portion sizes have increased over the years. Here's a novel idea: Try not eating out as much. But, when eating away from home, you can make special requests. Ask them to grill without butter or sauces. Split a meal, and put it on two plates for you and your partner. Ask for a doggy bag, and have them put half your meal in it before they bring it to the table.

FOOD FACTS

One of the main problems with diets is that most of them assume we have some sort of control over our days. Any working woman or mother knows that even with the best intentions, many meals are going to be eaten on the run and many others eaten in restaurants. Our eating patterns have changed, just since we were growing up. The amount of money we spend eating out has doubled since the 1970s. Fast food makes it so easy. And has anyone noticed the size of a burger since you were a kid? What about the size of a box of candy at the movies? Even the serving of broiled salmon they serve at the finest restaurants is big enough for two grown men to make a meal. We don't always know where we'll be eating our next meal, but it is almost a guarantee that we will be served more than we need.

WHAT ABOUT WILLPOWER?

It would be easy to just say, Well, I'll just eat less. I can control myself.

But it's more complicated than that. Willpower alone isn't the answer. What we eat and how our bodies metabolize the food are what really make the difference. To lose the jiggly fat squishing over the waist of your jeans and add firm muscle, you need to eat the right types of food, in the right amounts, at the right times. If you're thinking that sounds suspiciously like a diet, don't worry. You'll be eating so many different kinds of foods so often, you can even give the willpower a rest. A constant state of self-denial is no way to go through life.

Willpower alone isn't the answer.

WHAT HAVE WE BEEN EATING?

As a society, we decided that it seemed logical to cut the fat out of our diets if we wanted to lose fat. Unfortunately, while we were cutting back on fat, we also cut back on high-quality protein — lean meats, dairy, and eggs. In their place we added low-fat, high-carbohydrate foods that are easier to pick up like crackers, cookies, bread, chips, granola bars and muffins.

Instead of eggs in the morning, we have been eating bagels, sugary granola or buttery croissants. Dinners tend to be pastas or casseroles with garlic bread on the side. We may have a low-fat marinara sauce and a small salad on the side, but we are flooding our diet with the real culprit — refined carbohydrates.

Now we're not recommending a diet heavy in steak and dairy. What we advocate is a healthful combination of the right kind of foods — complex carbohydrates from whole grains, fruits and vegetables, and lean proteins, like chicken and fish. And as for the things you really love to eat, we would never tell you to completely deny yourself. We'll just show you ways to keep those foods in our life sensible. And we'll show you ways to substitute good foods for bad ones, without feeling ripped off.

TIMING IS EVERYTHING

The hardest concept to grasp may be that rather than eating less often, you need to eat more frequently. I think of your body as a furnace. You need to keep it consistently stoked with fuel. If you let it burn down to embers and dump a bunch of fuel on it, you get a lot of smoke and a big blaze, but soon you are right back where you started. If you add fuel consistently, you keep the fire burning steadily and cleanly.

So eat smaller meals throughout the day — 5 or 6 meals a day. This constant stream of energy will rev up your metabolism, and you will see how much better you feel. You know when you get cranky because your blood sugar gets low? Eating six little meals will help regulate your blood sugar. If you eat only once or twice daily, your body isn't sure when it will get fed next. It is more likely to store what it gets as fat because fat is our long-term energy storage. Eating more frequently makes your body use the calories more efficiently, and your energy level will go up. In fact, you could eat more calories in six small meals than in two large ones and actually lose weight. The fact is, you need fuel, and you need it all day long if your body and your mind are going to function optimally.

HOW WILL YOU KNOW WHAT TO EAT?

We said it before, and we'll say it again: This is not a diet. What we are describing is a system of eating based on your choices and your lifestyle. If you have specific dietary needs, please work with a nutritionist who is trained to address your unique issues regarding your diet. Let's talk a little about the different components of food and how our bodies react to them, so you'll know what to look for when you are making choices. Then we'll show you how we choose to make it work for us, then offer ideas of how it can work in your life. These facts are fascinating, and we encourage you to do further reading on your own and to consult with a nutritionist if you want even more specific information.

CARBOHYDRATES

Carbohydrates are the body's main source of fuel. Easily broken down by the body, carbohydrates give us the quickest surge of energy and are burned up by our bodies the fastest. They are what most of us crave when we are starving, sad, bored, or tired. There are good carbohydrates and bad carbohydrates. The bad ones are easy to identify — cake, candy, white bread — but even seemingly innocent foods like white rice and pasta are simple carbohydrates that break down just as quickly as candy, causing your mood and your energy to spike and surge, rather than remain consistent.

To make the situation worse, the effects of eating simple carbohydrates (the bad guys) don't just end when you finish the bag of chips or the beignets. As soon as your body burns through the simple carbohydrates you feed it, it crashes. What it wants is a quick fix — a dose of —that's right — simpler carbohydrates. How many times have you eaten one cookie and put the bag back, only to go back to the pantry several times for just one more until the bag is empty?

Carbohydrate craving on a repeated basis can strongly resemble an addiction, and is a very real fact of biology and metabolism, one which mere willpower is helpless to combat. Besides giving us that quick energy fix, carbohydrates are mood enhancers. The more sugary and starchy foods you eat, especially "comfort foods" such as chocolate cake, fried potatoes, frozen yogurt, the more the "feel good" brain chemical, serotonin, is released. Serotonin provides a calming effect, diffusing negative emotions like anger, depression and confusion. You feel rewarded, and you keep coming back for more.

Refined sugar is in almost all processed foods. It often comes in the form of high-fructose corn syrup (HFCS). Studies have shown that Americans have increasingly gained weight as a population since HFCS has been added to foods in the last 25 years. Additionally, it inhibits the brain's ability to feel full. You tend to eat more. We believe that reading food labels is one of the first steps towards loving your body. If HFCS is one of the first two ingredients, put it down and find a more natural food.

About 75 percent of us are genetically programmed so our bodies make excess insulin when we eat too many refined carbohydrates. About one-quarter of the population, has an extreme reaction to excess blood sugar — especially African-American, Polynesian, and Native American women. Another quarter of the population has few problems whatsoever with carbohydrates. These lucky souls don't understand how difficult it is for some of us to eat just one chip or cookie, because carbohydrates don't cause their bodies to secrete excess insulin. But the rest

of us need to stay completely off the carbohydrate roller coaster. Since our bodies need carbohydrates to function, the trick is to identify which ones are the good guys.

So what is a good carbohydrate? A complex, unprocessed carbohydrate takes longer to be used by the body. It releases its energy more slowly and doesn't cause insulin and energy surges. Beans, high-fiber cereal, oatmeal, whole grain breads, fruits and vegetables all contain the carbohydrates that our bodies need, but our bodies have to work for them so they won't put us on the roller coaster. We'll give you lots of specific examples of good carbohydrates, but the main thing to remember is that whole foods digest more slowly than refined ones.

Let's talk about how this happens. When you digest food, it turns into glucose. Glucose is what the fuel cells burn for energy. When we say blood sugar levels, we mean the amount of glucose circulating in the system. When your glucose levels drop too low, you feel dizzy, groggy and tired — low energy and no motivation. When blood sugar levels spike, your pancreas secretes insulin, which sweeps that sugar out of your system. When there is too much sugar and insulin can't do its normal job, it routes that extra sugar to your liver. Once that glucose gets to your liver, it is converted to fat, and you pack on the pounds.

This situation wouldn't be so bad if it only meant you were just a little chubby. The real problem is that over time,

ALTHOUGH THERE ARE MANY WAYS TO SABOTAGE YOUR HEALTH THROUGH POOR NUTRITION, WE BELIEVE THAT REFINED SUGAR IS PUBLIC ENEMY NUMBER ONE.

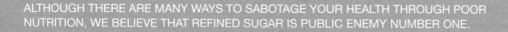

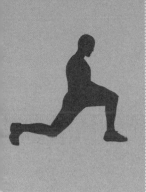

excess insulin in your system leads to overproduction of free radicals, which can cause damage to the blood vessels of your heart, leading to hypertension and high cholesterol — conditions that set you up for heart disease. Although most women think that breast cancer is a more serious threat to women, 1 in 27 female deaths are caused by breast cancer while 1 in 2 is caused by heart disease, the number 1 killer of women in the U.S. So keeping our carbohydrate input steady, choosing good ones and avoiding insulin spikes, is one of the important aspects of our plan.

PROTEIN

While carbohydrates are the body's fuel, protein provides the building blocks. Most women we meet just don't get enough protein. It is essential for the growth and repair of every cell in your body. Protein also builds strong bones, rich blood, healthy hair and nails, and it makes up the vital components for properly functioning immunity and digestion. Protein just makes you feel better, because it's the prime source of tyrosine, an amino acid which increases the production of brain chemicals that help you feel mentally sharp and alert. Protein subdues hunger pains more than fat and carbs and can help you reduce calorie intake.

But protein's key role in getting you fit is moving you away from fat-storing and toward the fat-burning mode. How can a food make you lose weight more efficiently? Glucagons. Protein foods stimulate glucagons — the fat-burning hormone that releases accumulated fats and makes them available to your body as fuel.

Think of glucagon as having the opposite job of insulin — it mobilizes or "spends" the glucose stored as fat in your fat cells, moving it to the muscles to be burned for fuel. When you eat lots of sugars and refined carbohydrates, you are elevating insulin levels which suppress your glucagon reaction. This makes it difficult for you to lose weight at a steady rate or to keep it off if you can lose it. A high-protein meal causes the slightest rise in blood glucose and a very small rise in insulin, but a significant increase in the glucagon level, and you start burning fat instead of glucose.

There are many sources of protein, so it's easy to find it in foods you like. Meat, eggs, fish, beans, nuts, seeds, and dairy products are all great sources of protein. As an aid to weight loss, protein fills you up faster, which can help reduce caloric intake. For most of us, it takes only 100 calories of protein to knock out our hunger pangs. While we could easily eat 1,000 or more calories of carbohydrates in a day, it would be difficult to consume

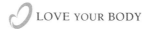

more than 700 calories of protein in a day. It would feel like you were stuffing your face in a pie-eating contest.

FAT

You probably have heard again and again that a high-fat diet is the culprit behind the alarming increase in obesity and disease in our country, but as we said before, this just isn't so. In a review of the medical studies on low-fat diets published in the New England Journal of Medicine recently, top nutritional researchers concluded that there is no apparent relationship between dietary fat intake and conditions such as obesity, heart disease and cancer.

It's a well-known fact that a whole-foods-based vegetarian diet naturally low in fat is extremely beneficial for you. But we can't emphasize this point enough — it's not fat that makes you fat, but eating a diet high in refined, simple carbohydrate foods and low in protein. That puts the pounds on and keeps them there. Of course, if you eat anything in excess, including fat, it's going to pack on the pounds, but one of the major steps towards loving your body is having a balanced approach in all areas of your life.

Fat can be your friend. It's hard to believe, but recent research shows that eating the right kinds of fats in the right proportions with other foods will actually help you control your weight more than if you cut fat out entirely. Eating moderate amounts of dietary fat will slow the digestion rate, allowing you to continue to feel full even after the proteins and carbohydrates have left the stomach. Another benefit is the way certain kinds of "friendly" fats are metabolized to impact insulin levels, to regulate blood sugar and the storage of fat.

What are these beneficial "friendly" fats that can aid in weight loss? Like carbohydrates, all fats are not created equal, and it's important to know which fats to eat in what quantities in order to make fat work for you, not against you. Let's talk about the various kinds of fats and the terminology used to describe them. Fats are classified by how solid they are at room temperature.

- Saturated fat – a solid; is butter, the marbled fat in beef, and coconut oil
- Unsaturated fat – a liquid (at room temperature); comes mainly from plant sources such as corn and safflower, and some fish
- Monounsaturated fat – the healthiest kind; is olive and canola oil; also found in avocado and almonds
- Polyunsaturated fat – corn, soy, and safflower oils; not as healthful as monounsaturated fats because of the kinds of essential fatty acids they contain.

Essential Fatty Acids (EFAs) have many important roles in our bodies. They are responsible for the formation of healthy cell membranes, the proper development and functioning of the brain and nervous system, proper thyroid and adrenal, the production of hormones, the regulation of blood pressure, liver function, immune responses, blood clotting, the breakdown and transportation of cholesterol and the support of healthy skin and hair. They're called essential because we need to take them in with the food we eat. Vitamins E, A, and D rely on fatty acids for their absorption and circulation throughout the body. There are a total of eight essential fatty acids that fall into two classes — omega-6 and omega-3.

A balanced diet supplies both omega-6 and omega-3. Omega-6 is found mainly in vegetable oils, and omega-3 comes from certain kinds of fish. The ratio of omega-6 oils to omega-3 oils should be about two to one, but in our modern diet with its refined foods, the ratio is usually off. We tend to eat ten times more omega-6 than omega-3 fatty acids. This imbalance makes our cells more susceptible to insulin resistance and high triglycerides (blood fat), both risk factors for obesity and heart disease.

To get your EFAs in balance and improve glucose tolerance, increase omega-3 intake. You can do this by eating deep-water fish like salmon, tuna, cod, or mackerel (preferably wild caught or from reliable sources to avoid metal contamination) two times a week, adding freshly ground flaxseed to your cereal, eating eggs, or including walnuts in your diet. In order to reduce your consumption of omega-6 fatty acids, avoid vegetable oils like corn and soy that can also suppress your metabolic rate. To increase your absorption of omega-3 fatty acids, make sure you take your B vitamins, magnesium, zinc, and vitamin C. You can find this combination available in any good multivitamin and mineral pill.

When oil is an ingredient, use olive oil and coconut oil, but use butter sparingly. Avoid hydrogenated and partially hydrogenated oils, which are chemically processed to increase commercial shelf life and contain damaging trans-fatty acids, which further throw off the EFA balance. The saturated fat of butter, eaten in moderation, is actually healthier than margarine. Reduce your intake of fried foods, vegetable shortening, many microwavable and TV dinners, crackers, cookies, cakes, and other convenience foods, and you'll be on your way towards eliminating harmful fats from your diet. If you haven't already, learn to use and appreciate olive oil, especially cold-pressed, extra-virgin olive oil that has undergone the least processing and

has the best taste. The healthy monounsaturated fats in olive oil do not produce trans-fatty acids when heated for cooking, and they resist rancidity when stored on the shelf.

Remember that there is no healthy level of trans fat. Studies have shown that people who eat about 4 grams of trans fat every day have a heart attack risk that is three times greater than people who eat about 2 ½ grams. Four grams of trans fat are in just one serving of fries from a fast-food restaurant. Trans fat makes your arteries less flexible and clogs them. It also reduces the good cholesterol — the HDL that sweeps through your arteries, virtually cleaning them out — and increases the bad cholesterol — the sticky LDL that gums up the arterial pathways and leaves you more susceptible to heart diseases. You will be able to find many of your favorite foods in versions that have no trans fat. They even make Fritos and Doritos without it these days. If you grew up in the Count Chocula era, however, there are some snack foods that you'll just have to forgo. The perils of trans fat are just not worth it.

FIBER

Getting enough fiber in your diet is also key to losing fat. As part of the plant foods that move food through the digestive system-fiber benefits us in many ways. It absorbs water and makes your bowel movements easier. It makes our digestive system generally healthier, improves our glucose tolerance and insulin response. It increases our feelings of being full, helping us to not overeat. In addition to helping us with our fat-loss goals, fiber is beneficial in reducing high blood pressure and other coronary heart disease risk factors as well as reducing the risks of developing some cancers.

Although current research indicates that we should eat 20-35 grams of dietary fiber every day, most of us get only between 12 and 18 grams. Fiber can be found in all plant foods to some degree. Beans, grains, vegetables (especially broccoli and carrots), some fruits and juices (particularly prunes, plums and berries), and root vegetables (like potatoes, sweet potatoes and onions) are all good sources.

Some types of fiber are not digestible until they reach the large intestine. They are called insoluble fiber. Sources of this type of fiber are whole grain foods, bran, nuts and seeds, vegetables — such as green beans, cauliflower, zucchini, and celery — and the skins of some fruits, including tomatoes. Think of fiber as your good friend who will not only fill you up, but also clean up after you.

WATER

No cleanup job is possible without lots of water. Although researchers are debating it, we feel strongly that it is important to drink large quantities of water — for your health and to lose fat. It is hard for us to distinguish between the feelings of hunger and thirst. Most of the time when we feel hungry, it is just our chronic dehydration crying out. Whenever you feel hungry, drink a glass of water and wait twenty minutes or so. Chances are, you weren't really hungry. Drinking water also keeps you from drinking other things, such as sodas — which have a whole slew of sins — and caffeinated beverages, which can further dehydrate you and make you hungrier. Caffeine is a diuretic, so it takes away more water from your system than it adds.

Water is also an important nutrient. It's vital for a many of our bodies' important functions, including removal of waste products, carrying nutrients, and regulating our temperature. Adequate intake of water also prevents fluid retention and helps us look less puffy.

To calculate how much water you need to drink every day, take your weight in pounds and divide by two. The result is the number of ounces of water you should drink a day. So a 140-pound woman needs to drink 70 ounces of water each day — at least six big glasses. It is just as important to drink water in the winter as it is in the summer. Your body uses water to stay warm, just like it needs it to make sweat and cool you off.

If you don't like the taste of plain water, try adding a little bit of lemon or lime. Some people can get more water down if it is ice-cold, while others prefer room temperature. Decaffeinated tea is also a good beverage, and hot tea has the added benefit of making you feel satisfied and full. Experiment until you find a way to get plenty of unsweetened, decaffeinated liquids into your system.

PUTTING IT ALL TOGETHER

Now you have the basics to get your eating in line with your goals. What a lot of information. How do you put it together? One of the reasons we were always frustrated with diets, even if they contained the same foods that we advocate, was that they were just so bossy and limiting. Neither of us likes to be told what to do, and even if we had wanted to eat these things just when they told us to eat them, we never seemed to be in the right place with the right food at the right time. We'll give you the formula here, and then show you how each of us puts our foods together. The way you fill in the blanks will depend on your own tastes and schedule.

Perhaps the most important thing you can do to make your eating work for you instead of against you is to write it down. We hear you groaning, but there's no way around it. If you don't track your food, you'll have no way of knowing what you actually ate. If you don't know what you ate, you won't know how to recreate what works for you. Perhaps most importantly, if you don't bring your food choices into the front of your mind — your conscious mind — you will still be eating from habit. Changing the habits that have gotten you out of shape and overweight is our whole goal here.

We have included a Food Journal in the back of this book (page 123) that you can reproduce on the copier, or you can get a little notebook and make your own. Whatever method of journaling you choose, you need to keep it with you in your purse, and keep it current. It is easy to believe that you will remember what you ate all day and write it down when you get home, but when you get home and your child has lost her homework, or you need to catch the dog that has gotten loose, you just tend to forget. We used to think that we could recreate entire days of eating, but we finally realized that we tended to remember the highlights — the perfect days or the terrible splurges,

rather than the solid regular days that were working us towards our goal. And if you haven't jotted your food down in a day or two, it is easier to blow it off than if you are faithful about keeping it. When a woman works out with a personal trainer, one of the top indicators that she will successfully meet her fitness goals is her ability to keep a consistent food journal. That should be good motivation to just do it!

OK. You've decided how to write down your food notes. You'll need space for seven days. Within those seven days, you'll need to eat every three hours, about six times during the course of the day. Remember that these are not six meals that are as large as the meals you have been eating, and you cannot skip them if you aren't hungry right then. It is important to keep adding the right fuel to your system so it burns off fat in the most efficient manner possible. Each little meal needs to include some protein, and during the course of the day you need to get your 5-7 servings of fruits and vegetables for vitamins and fiber. Make wise choices with your carbohydrates, and don't forget to drink that water. Put it on your chart, too, so you can keep track of it.

And don't worry: This all takes more effort to describe than it does to do.

89

BETHANY'S FOOD CHOICES

Breakfast (First Meal)

Breakfast is non-negotiable. No matter how grumpy or busy I might be in the morning, I make myself eat it. It gets the fire going, kick-starting my metabolism. I eat breakfast about an hour after I wake up, but I immediately have coffee with whole milk, and instead of real sugar, I use a vanilla-flavored, sugar-free syrup by Torani. I'd have cream if it were in the house! If you like the taste or consistency of skim or low-fat milk, that's fine, but I'm not skimping on my first taste of the day. That little indulgence puts me in a satisfied frame of mind and helps keep me from having cravings later in the day.

90

When I sit down to breakfast, or grab it to go, I choose one carb and one protein. I watch my portion sizes loosely. If you have been seriously involved in dieting at any point in your life like I have, you know those portion sizes by heart, but if you don't, we've put an easy table in the back of the book (page 120), and you can use food labels for reference. I try to eat about 200-300 calories at each small meal, but I don't stress over being exact.

Here are some proteins that are good at breakfast time. Try to get some variety in your breakfasts — so that you get a balance of nutrients, and so you don't get sick of eating the same thing every day.

Eggs: What a great source of protein and nutrients. There are so many ways to cook them. Scramble or poach one with a little butter and salt, make an egg white omelet with loads of vegetables left over from last night's dinner salad, or just keep a bowl of hardboiled eggs unpeeled in the refrigerator. When you need to run out in a hurry, it's ready to go. One is easily eaten in the span of one red light or a carpool stop.

Bacon: One piece of turkey bacon is good protein. When I started eating this way, I would even eat two pieces; but as I started seeing results, I began to eat just one. When you do buy bacon, look for the brands that are produced naturally or without nitrates. You can also find brands that offer lean-cuts. Always check the label if you are eating pre-cooked or frozen bacon.

Sausage: Look for lean meats or vegetarian sausage. There are lots of good frozen chicken sausages on the market now, and some grocery stores make store-brand sausages with interesting flavors. The spiciness of the sausage makes it fun and adds to that all-important feeling of satisfaction.

Cottage Cheese: I had always heard that cottage cheese was the perfect protein, and when I started to use the Love Your Body Fitness eating plan, I quickly understood why. You can make it savory or sweet, depending on your mood. You can add fruit and cinnamon, or vegetable and spices like chili powder or curry. It is very filling and contains great calcium.

Yogurt: Regular yogurt is high in carbs and sugar, so I go with Greek yogurt. I particularly like the Fagé Lowfat. It has good protein, and I mix with one or all of the following — vanilla, nutmeg, pumpkin pie spice, cinnamon. I top it off with a whole grain cereal and fruit, or sometimes I mix in canned pumpkin for the taste and fiber.

Along with my protein, I choose a carb. Here are some that work for me at breakfast time.

Oatmeal: This has never been my favorite, but I know how good it is for me, so I give it a try now and then. I make my own, because the instant packets are usually high in sugar, and the oats are not whole. There are many brands of oatmeal out there, but look for one that has steel cut or whole oats. The Silver Palate makes one that cooks relatively quickly. Sometimes I add walnuts, pistachios or pecans and a few raisins. Or, I'll chop up half an apple and add it to the mix. Cinnamon and other spices with a little Splenda or a dab of maple syrup keep it from having the high sugar content of the flavored packets, and it's just as tasty. You can add milk or yogurt on top, and you'll have protein and carbs all in one.

Cereal: I look for whole grain cereals like Fiber 1, Kashi, Grapenuts, 40-30-30 cereal, Ezekiel 4:9 Cereal and Shredded Wheat. I like to add fruit and nuts like almonds or walnuts. The important thing is to experiment and find what you like. Mix the cereals together for fun, and add nuts, fruit, or yogurt, and always watch your portions. Milk will complete your meal and give you more all-important calcium, as well as more protein. Although I do splurge on whole milk for my coffee, when I use milk with cereal, I can't tell the difference between whole and low-fat, so I save the fat and calories and go low!

Muffins: Most muffins are laden with fats and sugars. But VitaMuffin Vita Tops (www.vitalicious.com) are great. They have only 100 calories, 4-7grams of fiber, and 3-4 grams of protein. When I choose these muffins for breakfast, I also add a little more protein from milk, yogurt or meat.

Protein Shake: It's always better to eat real food, but sometimes it's easier to mix a shake. Just put some fruit, milk, ice and protein powder together and blend. Some companies offer the pre-made shakes. I use the Myoplex Lite Carb Sense Protein Shakes, and I mix them in a special way: I use a cup of fat-free milk and a half teaspoon of vanilla and shake it up before I add a little ice and blend. Although we believe that it is always better to eat whole foods whenever you can, getting the nutrition you need from a shake like this is better than not refueling at all.

91

Sometimes our mornings get so crazy, I just need to grab something that gives me my protein and my carb as I'm running out the door. Whole-wheat English muffins with a smear of peanut butter are quick to fix, as are whole-grain frozen waffles. Sometimes, I put walnuts and whole grain cereal with some raisins in a little Ziploc bag and make a little urban gorp. I go heavier on the nuts and lighter on the sugary dried fruit to keep the carbohydrate level down and make it as high in protein as possible. Nutrition bars are also great for those mornings when there isn't a moment to spare.

There are so many nutrition bars on the market, and so many of them are laden with sugar. You have to take the time to study the labels to see what is really in them. Try different brands. They all have different textures and consistencies, as well as different flavors. You will find several that you like. Look for bars that have at least 10 grams of protein and no more than 6 grams of sugar.

I like the Advantage Lite Carb Sense bars. Another new favorite is the Detour Bar Caramel Peanut — LOWER SUGAR (must say that on the label). It is great! I even eat this bar as a dessert. Some other bars I enjoy are Think Thin Creamy Peanut Butter bars and all the flavors of the Power Crunch bars. All these bars will have some sugar, but again, we are not into denial here, we are advocating making better, workable choices that will get us closer to our goals.

Mini Meal/Snack (Second Meal)

When I first started getting back into shape, I would wait until the standard lunchtime to eat again. As I continued my weight loss and became more in tune with my body, I realized I was getting hungry before lunch. I decided to eat some nuts as a snack. When lunchtime finally rolled around, I wasn't nearly as voracious as I had been. I also felt better. I noticed that as I increased the amount of my cardio-vascular exercise, I became hungry as soon as 30 minutes after a workout. When I asked Vince about this, he explained about "recovery food." To stabilize your blood sugar after working out, you need to eat healthy carbs and protein within 30 minutes. What a positive difference recovery food has made in my hunger and energy levels.

And I'll repeat this until you are sick of it, but don't forget to drink that water. Chances are, you're not as hungry as you think you are.

Snack choices

I like to pack a little cooler in the car if I know I am going to be on the go all day. I even carry small snacks that don't need refrigeration in my purse and the console of my car. If I always have a good choice on hand, I never fall into the trap of eating something of dubious nutritional value because it's the only thing available.

Nuts are always good choices, and a small handful is all I need to get enough protein. Almonds, walnuts, and cashews are all packed with nutrients as well as protein (and although they are high in fat, the fat is the healthy kind). Raw nuts are preferable to processed ones — roasted and salted nuts tend to be very high in sodium. I like soy nuts, too. When I get tired of the raw nuts, I spread out the raw nuts on a cookie sheet and roast them for about 15 minutes at 350 degrees. When I take them out, I rub a small pat of butter on the hot cookie sheet and add a little salt, chili powder, or other spices, and the nuts seem more like a treat.

Another one of my favorite snacks to add to my cooler is Mrs. Mays Cashew Crunch. She also makes a good Almond Crunch. Just four pieces (½ a serving) satisfies my sweet tooth and gives me a healthy form of protein.

An apple with a tablespoon of peanut butter or almond butter makes a great snack, as does a high-fiber, high-protein piece of bread with a smear of nut butter. There is one called "Men's Bread" that I particularly like, and there are others.

Lettuce leaves make great wraps. I add turkey and low-fat cheese, but any lean meat can make a good wrap. When I buy sliced meat, I try to find those that are naturally processed and don't have nitrates or MSG added as preservatives or flavor enhancers.

Low-fat or "Part-Skim" cheese sticks are a good source of protein and calcium, and with a small apple, they are a

satisfying snack. Olives are filled with healthy oil, and they can be a tasty snack. Cottage cheese or a low-fat yogurt like Fage with some fruit or carrot sticks is just as good as a snack as it was at breakfast time, and edamame (soybeans) is an easy source of protein.

Lunch (Meal 3)

When lunchtime arrives, whether I am still out running around or lunching with a friend, there are many choices that leave me feeling both satisfied and righteous. Some of my favorite lunch choices are bean soups — especially black bean.

I add avocado, bell pepper, onion, pico de gallo, or tomatoes. Sometimes, I add a teaspoon of shredded cheese or sour cream.

Grilled chicken salad is a great lunch option. When I first started eating consciously, I used a lot of salad dressing. As I have lost weight and begun to feel more and more energetic, I have begun to use less and less. Now I usually order dressing on the side and dip the tines of my fork in

93

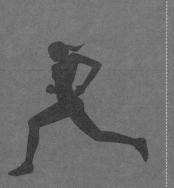

I LIKE LARA BARS, TOO. They don't have as much protein as the other bars I like, but with their whole-foods ingredients, they are very healthy. A little dab of almond butter tastes great on them and ups the protein level of my snack. I usually eat ½ a bar with a piece of fruit.

Whole wheat crackers like Triscuits, Dr. Kraker, or Kashi'sTLC with almond butter or low-fat cheese are always delicious, and Dr. Kracker even makes sweet ones called Graham Krackers which are delicious dipped in yogurt.

Two wedges of Laughing Cow Lite cheese with an apple are also great.

Greek yogurt is also a good base for a dip. Sometimes I mix it with sugar-free vanilla pudding as a dip for fruit. To make it a dip for veggies, I add garlic, onion, basil, or a Lipton soup mix like Onion or Spring Vegetable.

it. Sometimes I don't even feel the need for any dressing, but it took me some time to get my palate to the point where it could appreciate the very simple and unadorned taste of the food itself. On any salad, I always try to add as many vegetables as possible, for interest, vitamins and fiber.

I like salads made with grilled shrimp, salmon, or any fish in place of the chicken, too. The trick is just to avoid the fried stuff.

Turkey patties with cheese and pico de gallo are great. Low-fat beef patties are good occasionally, too. I like chicken salads made with a little vinaigrette or mustard, or plain low-fat yogurt instead of mayonnaise. Tuna salad made the same way is also a good lunch. I add pecans or cashews or, again, lots of vegetables. These salads can be served on sliced tomatoes, for extra nutrition and a lovely presentation.

Any grilled meat and vegetables is always a good choice for me. I just watch out for sauces that can be laden with sugars and fats. As with dressings for salad, I just ask for the sauce on the side and use enough to make the meal fun without sabotaging my goals.

Afternoon Snack (Meal 4)

Afternoon seems to bring an energy lull for most of us. Perhaps it is the busyness of the day, perhaps it is biorhythms, but without a doubt, low-blood sugar has a great deal to do with that feeling of exhaustion that can set in. Mid to late afternoon is a challenging time to make healthy eating choices, because our bodies are crying out for a little carbo satisfaction, and often kids are coming

home or being picked up to be taken to activities and are desperate for something to eat. To get through this danger zone, I remind myself to eat before I get ravenous, and I make sure and have some protein. A hot cup of decaffeinated green tea can hydrate me and put a warm cozy feeling in my stomach in the afternoon. My afternoon snacks are much the same as morning snacks, but I try to vary what I am eating so I don't get bored. Getting bored with my food, getting too hungry, and getting dehydrated are things I have to avoid to be happy and successful with the nutritional aspect of getting and staying in shape.

Dinner (Meal 5)

For dinner, my favorite choices are grilled, roasted or sautéed meats. I try to choose fish and chicken before beef. When I am out, I will even eat a hamburger, but I skip at least on half of the bun, or cut the burger in half. If I'm still hungry after half, I can eat the meat out of the other side with a fork.

I skip white potatoes and white rice. Wild rice is a good choice, and sweet potatoes are nutritional wonders. Squash is also a good substitute for starches, and gives me the same feelings of satisfaction. And vegetables are always a great choice — as long as they are not swimming in butter or cheese.

That is my basic food day. I don't obsess over totals, and I don't weigh and measure everything. I try to eat every three hours (or within 30 minutes of finishing a workout), and I make sure to have protein every time I eat. To train myself to eat consciously and to internalize these habits, I kept a food journal for a long time. Now, I am so familiar with the portions and food choices that work for me, that

I don't regularly keep a journal. If I find that I have gained more than two pounds, or if I am entering a period like the holidays when I know it will be easy to lose track, I will start journaling again until I am back on track.

I didn't decide to get in shape and immediately begin eating perfectly. I moved toward this style of eating in manageable increments. Every time I fell off the wagon, I just got back on. When I started seeing payoffs in my energy level and in the way my clothes fit, I got motivated to be a little more disciplined. Step by step, it was much easier to reach my goal than it had been all the times before when I was just trying to get there all at once and wondering why it never worked.

Those are my food choices, the variety that I can live with and enjoy. Look at how Vince makes his choices, and you can see how different personalities put it all together. Then you'll get a better idea of what will work for you.

95

96

VINCE'S FOOD CHOICES

Unlike Bethany, I don't mind having more structure in my food. My days are more predictable than hers, so I can schedule my meals pretty regularly. I also don't mind measuring and being precise — it's one of the things that keeps me on track and makes me feel that my food is working for me.

I get up early.

4:30 a.m. – Breakfast

1 serving steel cut oatmeal with fiber cereal, blueberries and ½ tsp agave nectar

2 patties or 2 links of vegetable sausage — I put a little olive oil on it because I like the flavor. I like the frozen Morning Star brand, and I just microwave it.

7 a.m. – Snack

Protein bar

½ Lara Bar

10 a.m.– Snack 2

Handful of Raw Nuts

Protein Bar

1 p.m.- Lunch

Almond butter sandwich on whole grain bread — 2 slices

I like the Men's Bread that Bethany likes, and I add some-sugar free jelly for that good PB&J taste.

Apple or pear

3:30 p.m. – Snack

Beef jerky

Nuts

Fruit of choice

6:30 p.m. – Dinner

Chicken – Grilled

Salad with balsamic vinaigrette dressing

Asparagus with olive oil

Like Bethany's, my food days vary, but the times I eat are consistent, and I don't tend to tire of foods as easily as she does. Unless I am eating out, what I've listed above is what I usually eat. When I do go out, I use the same guidelines she does to make the best choices possible. Having more healthy food choices makes it less necessary to keep a food journal regularly. If I get off-track, I will use one until I am back into good habits.

You know yourself best. You will know if you need to provide yourself with lots of choices and lots of flexibility or if, like me, you just want a program to stick with. Whichever route you choose, write it down until it becomes second nature. There are many theories about how long it takes to create a habit, but when it comes to food, it is always safer to err on the conservative side. Our food habits are rooted in our childhoods, before we were even making conscious decisions, and in our chemical makeup. Stick with the journaling until you are secure in your new habits. It takes at least three months to build a "new brain." Think of the journaling as training wheels — you'll get there just as fast using them, and you won't fall off as often!

Stress is something we cannot always control. Men and women in the thirty to sixty-age bracket have stress. It comes from children, divorce, sick parents, bad marriages. Stress alone can cause some women to hold

97

more fat. In fact the more stress you have can mean the more weight you put on. This happens because stress activates the "flight or fight" response which then makes the adrenal glands produce cortisol. This hormone makes the cells release energy that allows you to run (say from that wild animal!) or to fight. Even when the threat is gone, your level of coritsol stays raised. This is great when you need to outrun a bobcat, but day after day this can wreak havoc on your body. According to a study at the University of California at San Francisco, women who carry "excess weight" in their abdominal area "secreted significantly more cortisol than women who did not have extra belly fat." We all know that fat around the middle is toxic. What is even worse is that this need to refuel the tank makes our bodies think we are hungry, and we feel as if we need food. A terrible cycle if you ask me!

Do what you can to eliminate stress. Talk to your friends and family. See what alternate plans they can come up with.

Chapter 7

The Right Choices For Your Lifestyle

I ran into a friend I have known since our early 20s. She said, "I've known you for 20 years. You've never looked like this. You're a babe. Will you e-mail your diet?" When I sent it to her, I called it the Babe-a-liscious diet. But it wasn't just a diet; it was my new self. You may not be amazed at my story — I didn't go from 300 pounds to 115. I haven't done anything very different than what other healthy people do. I just found an easier way to do it.

The most important part of learning to love my body was being honest about who I am. I hate to deny myself! I have changed the way I eat and the way I think about fitness. Sure, the weight loss is great, but the most important thing is how good I feel and how much energy I have. I think about food in a completely different way than I used to.

Is it worth it? Absolutely! Most of the time fattening, sugary foods are just not worth it to me. I would rather stay strong and healthy. I have lost and kept off 40 pounds. My body fat is 19%. I feel good. I feel sexy. I feel strong! I like how my clothes look on me. At long last, I don't have to hold my stomach in. This way of eating and exercising makes me feel the best I have ever felt in my life.

I wish I had known in my 20s what I know now. This is one of the reasons I wrote this book. I have several friends who have watched me change my lifetime of bad habits. Some of them are recently out of college. They ask me how they can do it too. I try to tell them it really is easier for them because they have youth on their side. This book is for them, but it is also for my friends 40 and above. If I can do it, you can, too!

Most of the women I know these days don't have what I would call a lifestyle, they are just busy putting out fires most of the time. "Lifestyle" sounds so organized and controlled, like a vision in which all the children go up to bathe on their own at 5:00, and dinner is served promptly at 6. Throw in sports schedules, tutors, book clubs, volunteer meetings for yourself, volunteer meetings for your children, work commitments, work socializing, and hopefully a few friends, and lifestyle seems to have become a whirlwind of activity, blowing us from one event to the next. If we are lucky, we arrive at all these events somewhat on time, almost organized, and if we are really, really good, we will appear calm when we get there. But lots of us are just glad to make it on time to the next event, and, isn't it nice that they've served tasty snacks to make it special.

Who are these people that think they are doing us a favor by serving M&Ms, St. Andre Cheese, or donuts at all these non-party functions we all seem to be attending these days? It always seemed to me that everyone else was eating these yummy things without giving it a second thought, so why shouldn't I? There were times when I used to tell myself I deserved a treat for having gotten to this meeting at all. Other times, I was so tired from staying up late getting everything done and not eating enough good food during the day that I was just starving. Because of crazy living like that, I would have eaten anything that came within a three-foot radius of my mouth. While I can't tell you how to control the speed at which your world turns, I can give you some tips to make sure you don't deal with life's inevitable pressures by sneaking off down the carbo-loading trail. Let's look at some ways to make good choices during the busy week, and then what to do on the weekends that sometimes are more hectic.

I'll just cut to the chase. For many women, one of the biggest challenges to fitness is wine. The research on wine is so confusing: Drink a glass of wine every day if you want to be heart-healthy and beautiful like a French woman. Don't drink wine if you have any history of breast cancer in your family (and who of us doesn't have some female relative who has been touched by breast cancer?). If you want to drink wine for your health, but you haven't started, then don't. Don't drink only on the weekends;

don't drink more than 4 ounces a night…just reading all the conflicting advice makes you want to have a drink. But you will have to wade through all that information on your own, because it is so personal to your body chemistry, your family history, and your lifestyle. Once you get all that figured out, and you still want to have that adult beverage, be smart about it.

There are many studies about the relationship of alcohol to blood sugar and weight gain. In terms of keeping my weight steady, I find only red wine, low-carb beer and an occasional cocktail with a diet drink work. Some studies say that there is no difference among the types of alcoholic beverages consumed, but I say no white wine. Skip the champagne, too, on a regular basis, but if someone opens a great bottle to celebrate, don't say no, just have a taste. It's all about balance.

The trimmer you get, the more you need to cut down on alcohol. I went from having a glass of wine five to six times a week to two or less. As I have gotten fitter, my focus has changed. I have more energy and am more relaxed, and the calories in alcohol aren't really worth it to me. I'm also able to get a better workout in if I skip the wine. When I do drink I always start with a glass of water before I have a glass of wine. Then I have two waters and then my second glass of wine. This keeps me hydrated as well as full, and I have that glass in my hand just like everybody else.

Once you get the wine situation under control, start looking at what is worth the calories to you. How do you motivate yourself to make good choices? Everyone has her own weakness. Although my willpower is getting stronger month-by-month, as we have said before, willpower is not what is going to get your weight down and keep it there.

You need to find ways to make peace with those foods — and drinks — that call out to you like sirens, dragging you to diet destruction. For me, queso was a huge problem. I used to take my children to a Mexican food restaurant and gorge on chips and queso. The children were happy, and I was comforting myself like crazy, until I realized that every time we went there, I was looking at the crumbs at the bottom of the second chip basket, feeling like a sick beached whale, and dinner hadn't even come out yet. But the next time we would go, there I went again.

I was bound and determined to get through it. I decided that I would keep going back to the same restaurant night after night until I could just skip the chips. The first night I felt like a very noble martyr, and while it worked, I couldn't have sustained that pose for very long, at least not happily. The second night I had the foresight to order a large bowl of the marinated carrot/onion mixture. I was able to drizzle a small amount of queso on my plate. I skipped the chips. The next night I skipped the queso all together. I have it now occasionally, but I am not addicted to it like I was.

We all have different quesos in our lives, and the trick is not to run away from them. Meet them head-on and realize that they are not putting themselves in your mouth, and they are not mesmerizing you. You are consciously deciding to eat them. While the strong desire to eat them is probably from further back in your mind, you control the action. Face those trigger foods often enough that you can tell yourself you don't need to eat them right now. Right now. That's all. They will still be there tomorrow, or next week. And if you feel the need to placate someone's feelings by eating something special they have made for you, just have a little, tell them how great it was, and tell yourself that you can have some more later. Then throw or give the rest away when they are not looking. And if a little nagging voice inside tells you that it's a sin to waste food, recognize that little red-horned voice for the rationalization that it is and just say it's more of a sin to overindulge! No one but you should be in charge of the food choices you make.

Start by recognizing what foods have some sort of a grip on you, and break that hold by facing it. Then you can look at general categories of foods that aren't doing you any favors, and set some guidelines for yourself. Let's look at ways to deal with bread and desserts — two food categories we tend to find so comforting but can easily pack on the pounds.

BREADS AND DESSERTS

While queso was difficult for me in Mexican restaurants, white bread and desserts are trying to get me everywhere I go. Rather than trying to have a standoff with each of them, I developed what I call the Three-Bite Rule. I take three bites, as big as I wish (although sometimes I do have to remember to mind my manners because people are watching!). I also made an agreement with myself that I just wouldn't eat store-bought bread or desserts. When I eat these foods, I want the taste and the experience to be worth the calories. Store-bought cookies really don't taste as good as fresh-baked chocolate cookies hot out of the oven. If I told myself that I would never eat dessert or white bread, I would immediately start craving both of them. But with these gentle guidelines, I never feel deprived, but I also don't set my blood sugar racing.

I sometimes eat a piece of fruit before eating dessert. I also always try to drink a glass of water. Being a little full

helps with my sweet craving and makes three bites more than enough. Hot decaffeinated or herbal tea also gives me a feeling of satisfaction, and makes no dessert no big deal.

When you eat bread, make sure it is the whole grain variety. All bread is not created equal. Look at the label — there are those labels again — and check the order of ingredients. If whole grain flour is not the first ingredient, move on (and, of course, if partially hydrogenated vegetable oil is on the label at all, move away quickly). When you are having a sandwich, double the meat and halve the bread if you are using white bread. Or use lettuce to make a wrap out of your sandwich ingredients instead of bread. If you can't bring yourself to skip the roll yet, just take three bites. Eat your vegetable first, and get a little full before you start on that roll. Drink a glass of water before your meal comes if you are still craving more bread. Just as with dessert, don't tell yourself "No." You'll just see that forbidden fruit on the other side of the fence and crave it. Go up to it, taste it, and realize that there's nothing there that you're not going to have the opportunity to have some other time.

RESTAURANTS

Even though the FDA has told us that there is definitely a link between eating out and obesity, that doesn't seem to keeping anyone I know out of restaurants. We know what the culprits there are: portion size, hidden ingredients (oh, that lard in the salad dressing tastes good!), and the feeling that it's not a meal, it's a celebration. Well, eating at a restaurant might have been a celebration back in Laura Ingalls' day, but at this point, it's just a fact of life. And it's something we can deal with and enjoy without new pants or a girdle.

103

You can eat well and be satisfied at any restaurant. There are some general tricks, and some that are specific to restaurant type. In general, remember to order an appetizer as your main course. You save money and calories. You don't owe your waiter anything, and he is not going to think you are either fat or stingy if you do this. If you can't get past this waiter guilt, just tip him on the dinner-sized portion, and he'll forget anything bad you think he might have thought! Remember portions are crazy these days. The salad with all the dressing and candied walnuts and crumbled blue cheese could feed two or three people. Share it with your dinner companion if you want a starter, or get an extra side of veggies with your main course. Or do get a salad for entertainment and roughage before the meal, and get the dressing on the side. If you must have fries with your steak, three bites. And eat slowly. Put your fork down and visit with your dinner companions. If they are all toddlers, put your fork down and help them color their menus. Give your body time to feel full; not only will you enjoy your meal more, but also you will not be tempted to overeat. Eating should be about two things — refueling your body and breaking bread with those you love (or do business with). While the sensuality of food and the experience has an entire culture that has been built up around it, you can have those experiences without jeopardizing your health. Remember, the chocolate bonbon that is presented to you at the end of a special meal is not the only chocolate bonbon that you will ever encounter. If you're full, if you've had three bites of dessert, if feeling great is more important to you than tasting it, just say no thank you (with no explanation) and tell yourself you will have it next time. Food will not make our mothers love us more, make us powerful, take away any sadness, or do

anything but put calories and nutrition in our bodies. By all means, enjoy your experience in the restaurant, but don't use it as an excuse to overeat. Here are some ways I've learned to happily and healthily navigate different types of restaurants:

MEXICAN

Let's have a moment of silence for that queso that used to have me in its grip. But I've moved on, so I don't need to go back there. When I'm at a Mexican restaurant now, I eat a lot of beans, fajita meat without the tortillas, or one taco with double meat. Guacamole is high fat, but high in nutritional value and very satisfying. I love to order ceviche if they have it, and many Mexican restaurants now have some grilled shrimp and fish dishes. I try to remember to ask them to lighten the cheese, and I add flavor with salsa instead. I skip the refried beans and ask for the charro beans or any whole beans instead. Black bean soup or chicken tortilla soup are good choices, and I just make sure not to smother either with cheese.

ASIAN

When they offer chopsticks, I take them. It is very difficult to overeat with chopsticks, because they just don't hold that much. I am invariably full before I have gotten the whole meal up to my mouth. I love Vietnamese, Thai, Chinese and Japanese food. If you skip the tempura, most of what is in Asian food is protein and vegetables. If it's not already, sushi should become your friend. Japanese restaurants usually have great salads, too. I even have skewers of grilled shrimp. Miso soup is high in protein and is great for you. Try it. You might fall in love with it. Sashimi is a great option. Fried is not your friend. I think Chicken Lettuce wraps are super, and instead of ordering fried egg rolls, I order Spring rolls (fresh ingredients wrapped in rice paper). When I feel like I just have to have a little rice, I order brown rice. Hot and sour soup, wonton soup, and others are always a good start — warm, tasty, and, most of all, satisfying.

ITALIAN

When I think Italian, I include pizza joints. At other Italian restaurants that do have a varied menu, minestrone is a great starter. When I'm offered a side of pasta, I always ask if they can substitute veggies. Tomato sauce is always better than cream. If they serve whole wheat pasta, It Is always a better choice than white. Many restaurants will serve a piece of grilled chicken and put the sauce on the side. As long as the sauce is there, I don't move into that "poor me, so deprived" mode and try to cheer myself up with more food. And, try the spinach. Italian restaurants always make the best spinach.

FAST FOOD

Fast food can be tricky, but after the movie *Supersize Me,* even McDonald's has salads and healthier choices. If you go for a burger, eat half, or skip half the bun. Order it without mayo and without cheese. You won't notice, and several hundred calories will be saved. Can't resist those fries? Three should do you!

HOLIDAY MEALS

When you can finish a holiday meal full of love and affection for your family and still stick to your eating plan, not feeling deprived or guilty, you'll know you have really gotten your relationship with food to a good place. We all know how much work it can take to get any

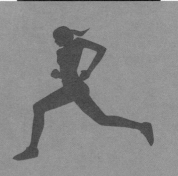

I REMEMBER DRIVING UP TO A PIZZA PLACE ON A FAMILY TRIP. I like pizza, but it isn't something I have ever craved like some of my friends. As we pulled up my husband asked me to pop out and see if they had something on the menu I would eat. They did have a green salad, but it was limited. When I suggested another spot, my kids asked when I was going to be "normal" again. When I told my friends this story they said, "Awww" – not like how cute, but like how sad. But Vince said "Bravo." He got it. My kids are regular kids. They get all the junk food marketed to them. But now, they're learning through example. Here's how the story ended: We went in. We ordered thin crust rather than thick. I asked for extra veggies and to go light on the cheese. It was all really normal, and also healthy.

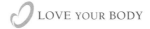

relationship to a good place, but here are some things that help me at Thanksgiving and other significant holiday meals.

First, tell yourself that you plan to be around next Thanksgiving. Chances are, if your family is like most, next Thanksgiving will dawn with the same array of pecan and pumpkin pies, green bean casseroles, rolls, cranberry sauce — all the favorites. Yes, they only come out once a year, but they will be back next year, and you will enjoy them much more if you are not stuffed. Eat a little of everything you like, but focus on the turkey or meat, and any vegetables that you can find that are not drowned in cream of mushroom soup. And, of course, have some pie. Three bites.

Don't make a big announcement about how hard you are trying to "be good," or chances are a host of relatives will set in on you, either trying to tempt you to join their ranks and overindulge, or making such a fuss about how good you are that you'll start focusing too much on the food. Remind yourself that the food tastes much better when you eat enough slowly than when you eat too much too fast. Remember Mary Poppins: "Enough is as good as a feast." And if someone notices that you are not gorging with the rest of the crowd and starts in on that old "It only

comes once a year; live a little" stuff, just smile, raise your glass and say, "Eat up! It's delicious, but I am just full." Tell yourself that yes, Thanksgiving only comes once a year, but there's always Christmas, Hanukkah, New Year's, Valentine's Day, Easter, Sunday lunch, your birthday, your family's birthdays, your coworkers' birthdays, Flag Day, Mother's Day, Veterans Day, Memorial Day…you get the picture. You're not going to be deprived, and you just might find yourself feeling fitter and looking better by the time next Thanksgiving comes around.

PARTIES

Parties, of course, have their own special challenges. Some parties are all about being with friends, but there are also lots of parties where we feel we need to put our best foot forward, and it can be a little nerve-wracking. And what do we want to do when we feel a little nerve-wracked? That's right — we eat a little something to take the edge off, or to give us something to do when we don't see anyone we know, or we cozy up with that glass of wine.

So go prepared. First, never go to a party hungry. If you are too focused on getting your nutritional needs met, you won't have time to really enjoy the festivities and the other friends. Before you go, have a protein snack and a glass of water. Slip a protein bar into your evening bag. At the party, have another glass of water before you order a cocktail.

If you are at a buffet, get a small plate and fill it with veggies, meat, and three bites of festive food. When you are done, put your plate down, pop a breath mint, and find someone new to talk to or something else to do. If it is a sit-down dinner, just eat smart. If the salad is heavily

106

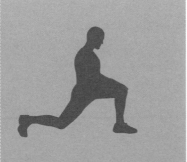

LITTLE HABITS LIKE BREATH MINTS SIGNAL TO YOUR BRAIN THAT IT IS FINISHED EATING. I brush my teeth after dinner to tell myself that I am done eating for the day.

dressed, three bites. If the hostess says, "Oh, you must have more," remind her that you are saving room for what is to come. Remember that people are trained to push food on you. They do it with the best intentions, but it is up to you to say no. You can show your appreciation of their culinary skills and their efforts without eating yourself into a glassy-eyed stupor. Go heavy on the praise and light on the bites, and you will be fine.

And, make sure you don't drink too much. Besides adding lots of unnecessary calories, that alcohol will loosen your inhibitions — it won't make you any cuter or funnier, it will just make you crave carbohydrates and probably say things you'll wish you hadn't said the next morning. One drink will relax you and give you the fun party feeling. More won't do anything but get you into trouble — either with your scale, your husband or your friends. The time for bragging rights on hangovers and winning parties ended back in college, and don't we all wish they hadn't been part of the scene back then either? Party on, but party smart!

HUSBANDS AND SIGNIFICANT OTHERS

Husbands are not a type of meal, but they can influence our eating in so many ways that I think it's important to mention them. There are as many types of husbands as there are sizes of women, so I am not going to try to generalize except for three basic things.

1) Don't think you need your partner to eat what you eat. It is rare that a husband and a wife decide they want to focus on being fit at the same time. Usually, just when you want to hit it hard and have little salads and a bit of fish for dinner, your husband will start talking about steak or nachos. Or, the other way around, you have been resolutely disciplined, and you think you're just going to take a little break, and your husband stands up as Mr. Righteous Eater, across whose lips no simple carbohydrate has or will ever pass. You ask him if he wants to split a little Death by Chocolate because it's the night before your period and you just need your three bites to survive, and he looks at you like you have asked him to shoot heroin. While it is possible for you to support each other in your fitness and diet goals, it is important to remember that it doesn't matter what your husband or partner eats. Some dogs are greyhounds; some dogs are St. Bernards; all dogs need specific amounts of food to be healthy. Somehow when it is dogs, it doesn't seem like such a judgment of worthiness or love, it's just a biological fact of how the dog is made. Well, it's the same with people. You need to eat what keeps you fit and healthy and satisfied, and tune out what anybody else is eating. And don't make any value judgments about what anyone else does or doesn't eat. You have no way of knowing what has crossed their lips during the day before you sat to dine with them.

2) I mentioned this before, but it is worth revisiting here, because it is so important: Don't decide to get fit because you think your husband wants you to, or because you think any romantic and/or life partner would love you more if you were trimmer. Loving your body means YOU loving your body. Sometimes it is hard to separate the approval of those we love from our own inner feelings of what we want and our confidence level, but it is important to figure out the difference. Being fit is always something you do for yourself first

107

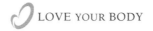

— for your health, for your positive self-image, and for your enjoyment of life. The people you live with will no doubt make comments about what you are eating as your habits change. Hopefully they will recognize that what you are doing is a positive thing for you.

Sometimes, however, people are not as secure as we think they are, and changes in the people they love threaten them. "What if she gets really fit and she dumps me?" or "What if she looks great, and I look like an old tub of lard beside her?" or even "I'm supposed to be the fit one around here." The list goes on, and while these may sound like exaggerated concepts, remember that food is the first form of nurture that any of us receive, and our feelings of being loved are often closely tied to our eating habits. Another response might be, "Why aren't you making me that fabulous German chocolate cake anymore? You must not love me. If you really loved me, you could make it and just not eat it…" You get the picture. Remember: food is food, and love is love, and while there are many occasions when both are present, they are two very different things. Don't let anyone convince you otherwise. Keep that in mind, and if you notice any significant other putting any type of pressure on you — either positive or negative — just remind yourself you are doing this for your well-being. If you need to love someone a little bit more, someone who is out of sorts, by all means do it, but you don't need to make unhealthy eating choices to show solidarity with anyone.

3) If the person you live with needs some help loving his body, lead by example. Start filling your pantry and refrigerator with healthier choices. Make gradual

improvements on the fare you serve. Talk about how much better you feel, but don't lecture or nag. Just as you needed to be the one to start loving your body, he needs to be the one to love his. It is amazing when you start seeing your success and can't believe how great you feel. You will want to tell everybody all the time. But temper your zeal with empathy, and remember how you felt before you started loving your body. You can show your husband — or your children — the path without dragging them down it.

VENTI, TEA OR ME?

Ever since the dawn of Martha Stewart, we have all realized that our lifestyle is not something to take for granted; it is something that can be improved. Improvement comes in many ways, and we are constantly being bombarded with language that tries to appeal to our sense of who we think we are (read that "who we think we ought to be"). Coffee is no longer the hot cup of Joe that it was in our parents' time. It is java, café, shade-grown or free-trade. It comes from places we might only dream of going to, and it speaks of greening the planet and saving society.

Advertisers have become so talented with nuanced pitches they make to us every minute of every day, that we don't notice most of them. Back to that cup of coffee: No matter how elegant or continental or "swav-A" that Venti sounds, all it means is Extra Large. Super-Sized. Put back into plain cuppa joe language, all it really means is nobody needs that much coffee at one time. Nobody needs 36 ounces of an all-fruit smoothie, no matter how many vitamins it has in it. All those fabulous milligrams of vitamin C and anti-oxidants and free-radical fighting phytonutrients, Amazon berry-health wizards all come hand-in-hand with bags of sugar — sometimes up to 56 grams! Can you imagine what 56 grams of sugar looks like? That's one big pixie stick that none of us needs to open. But the language just tells you about the health benefits, it doesn't mention the downside of the product.

It is up to us to see that flowery language for the manipulative marketing that it is. Venti, grande, super-sized, double-stuffed, con queso, all you can eat, dessert with meal — instead of thinking that these terms are getting you glamour, or a bargain, or whatever your self-image is drawn to, take those same words and apply them to your body. Super-sized? NO thank you! Double-stuffed? You get the picture. Once you start noticing how many ways unhealthy foods — and too much of them — are marketed to you, you will be amazed. And, more importantly, you will be able to buy the things you need when you need them. That is one of the most important lifestyle improvements you can ever make, and it sure feels good to down-size!

HYDRATE OR DIE

The last thing I want to address in this section about lifestyle is the importance of drinking lots of good, clean water. Once it was a very popular movie-star thing to have some kind of designer water in a special pouch. While that aspect of hydrating was just a silly fad, the underlying idea of drinking water throughout the day was quite sound. Experts disagree about how much you need daily. You can certainly read studies that will tell you to drink eight ounces eight times a day and to drink a full glass of water before every meal or after every alcoholic drink, and on and on. We need to drink water to flush out our organs,

to keep kidney stones from forming, to replace fluids that are lost when we sweat. If you are sedentary, sitting at the desk in the air-conditioning, of course you won't sweat so much. But if you are loving your body, you are getting out and moving it and sweating up a storm. You need to drink lots of water.

It is important to drink that water before you are thirsty. You need a glass of water when you get up, before you work out, while you work out, and after you work out. You need to take a sip from that fountain when you pass by. You need to drink water instead of sweetened or caffeinated beverages. You need to think of a long cool draught of water as cleansing you and filling you with goodness, the same way you feel a deep breath filling you with oxygen and carrying waste products away. Water is your friend, and whatever bottle you drink it in, whether you like it lukewarm or chilled, with lemon or lime, straight from the tap or from an exotic mineral spring, it is good for you, and it should be a big part of how you love your body.

THE FOOD JOURNAL IS YOUR FRIEND

The time has come to look at the food journal. Everything I have told you is easy to do, but sometimes getting it all together is a little daunting until it becomes a habit. As Vince and I have told you, some people need to use their journal religiously, or they just go crazy eating funnel cakes and forgetting all about it by the afternoon. Others just need to check in and journal for a few days or weeks when they find themselves slipping into too much rationalizing or other bad habits. Whichever camp you are in, or near, it is of the utmost importance to use a food journal until you develop good habits.

Some people say it takes 21 days to create a habit; who knows if that is true? Try the food journal for a month. If you do it the way we propose, you will definitely see results. If you do it but don't change your eating habits, at least you will immediately identify the culprits weighing you down. And if you can't figure out why pounds won't come off, the food journal is always the first place to start. It is an accurate record of what, how much, and how often you are eating, and if you're getting enough protein.

Here's what it looks like:

Date:			
MEAL	**Time of day**	**What did you eat?**	**Did you have protein? What was your mood?**
#1 (wake up)			
#2			
#3			
#4			
#5			
#6 (2-3 hours prior to bed)			

Keep it in your purse, and soon after you eat jot down what you ate. 7 almonds? Great. Also note the time you ate. Two scoops of lemon custard ice cream? Not so great, but make sure and write it down.

Here's an example of a week of Bethany's eating when she first started journaling. You'll notice how the food choices are not "perfect." If you aren't honest with yourself here, you will have no way of knowing how to improve.

It will take you a few weeks to see patterns in your eating, and we hope that as you go along, you will see improvements in your choices. Your journal is for you — not to impress yourself, not to berate you, but to be a record. Seeing things written down in one place is the only way to understand exactly what you put in your body. No record of the past, no hope for change in the future. Keep your food journals together in one place and when you have a month's worth, go through them. See what worked, what you were eating when you felt good. See what patterns emerge: Lots of parties? Vacation? Big gaps in your journal?

Food journaling will tell you about more than just what you eat, it will tell you about how much control you have over your life. Too busy to write down what you ate? Too busy. It is a simple yardstick, but committing to use it will add a sense of order to your life that will have benefits in other ways. Think of it as a lifestyle journal and a really honest friend.

Chapter 8
Tips and Tricks

112

Here are some quick reminders of things we have covered in depth earlier in the book. Look them over, and use them in the ways you think will be most helpful to you. You might choose one every day and write it on a Post-it where you'll be certain to see it. You might choose one each week and try to focus your week around it. Some will speak to you more loudly than others. See what works for you.

1. Get to the gym.
2. Add Strength Training to your workouts.
3. Exercise at least 4 times a week.
4. Even if you just get in a 30-minute workout – MAKE IT COUNT.
5. Do speed intervals or sprint your run! Push it.
6. Don't let your fun revolve around food.
7. Eat breakfast. Eat before you work out!
8. Get an extra hour of sleep. Lack of sleep increases the appetite.
9. Drink that water. Go for eight glasses today!
10. Eat small meals – Boost your metabolism in an easy way.
11. Put salt and pepper on your desserts after your three bites to prevent over-eating!
12. Put a photo of yourself in a bathing suit on your refrigerator.
13. Eat before the party – take food with you.
14. Plan ahead for the day. Keep healthy snacks, food and bottled water in your car, purse and briefcase.
15. Eat protein with every meal/snack. Protein makes you feel satisfied – especially with a bit of carbs and a bit of fat.
16. Split a meal at a restaurant.
17. Follow the Three-Bite Rule on bread and desserts.
18. Get rid of the junk food in your house.
19. Water/Wine/Water/Water/Wine.
20. Wean yourself – never go cold turkey on the things you like.
21. When you have eaten your last meal of the day, brush your teeth. This signals your brain that you are indeed done eating.
22. If you can afford only one session – get professional help from a trainer or fitness specialist.
23. Pick a group of foods that work for you. Always have these on hand. When you are in a rush, pick one! My grouping would be the following: ½ almond butter sandwich, cottage cheese, almonds, other nuts, protein, chicken breasts, a salad I love from a fast-food restaurant, apples with Laughing Cow lite, etc. When I am tired or in a rush, I know I can get one of these.
24. See this as a permanent change. Tell yourself I want to make my food choices so good that I can do this forever. This isn't just a way to lose weight. This is a way of life.
25. Love Your Body!

So that's it. You know all our secrets now, and you've probably realized that they aren't very secret or very technical. They are facts of life, tried and true ways of moving your body and fueling it that will leave you with a new feeling of satisfaction and contentment with your body — a real love and respect. We are not offering you a magic combination of foods that will sweep pounds away before your eyes. We want you to learn to love yourself and your body more than you love food. We want you to realize that the short-term pleasure of overindulgence never outweighs the long-term goal of feeling good. We want you to know that eating habits can be changed, and there are lots of good tricks to going about it. We hope you have found a great deal of useful information in these pages that will help you break up with those unhealthy foods and get tighter with yourself.

And as for exercise, we do run boot camps, and it is our job to help women, just like you, reach their fitness goals. But we want you to know that you don't have to be in a boot camp to get fit. You just need to move. What our boot camps have taught us is that doing it all alone is lonely.

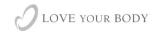
It's just not fun. Admitting that we want to be in shape and getting support to do it is the only way that we can stay healthy. We have to be honest with ourselves before we can say it out loud, but having the support of a friend once we say it out loud is the best way to love ourselves. Love takes place in community, and we are all trying to reach the same goals. We want to be healthy and happy. Sure, we've all taken lots of detours on the way, and events will probably come up in our lives again that will threaten to get us off the path, but if we set our sights firmly on loving our bodies, we will have the best chance of long-term success.

Cardiovascular exercise, resistance training and good eating habits — these are the three parts of our not-so-secret secret. We've shown you how we put them together, now it's time to get started. Remember that we're here for you. When you need new exercises, when you need motivation, when you need to know more, check the website. We offer all kinds of information and inspiration to help you love your body. If we can do it, you can do it. And you're going to love it!

114

LOVE YOUR BODY: THE SECRET TO SUCCESS!

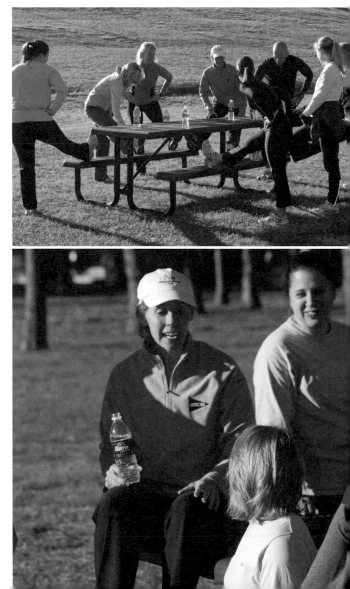

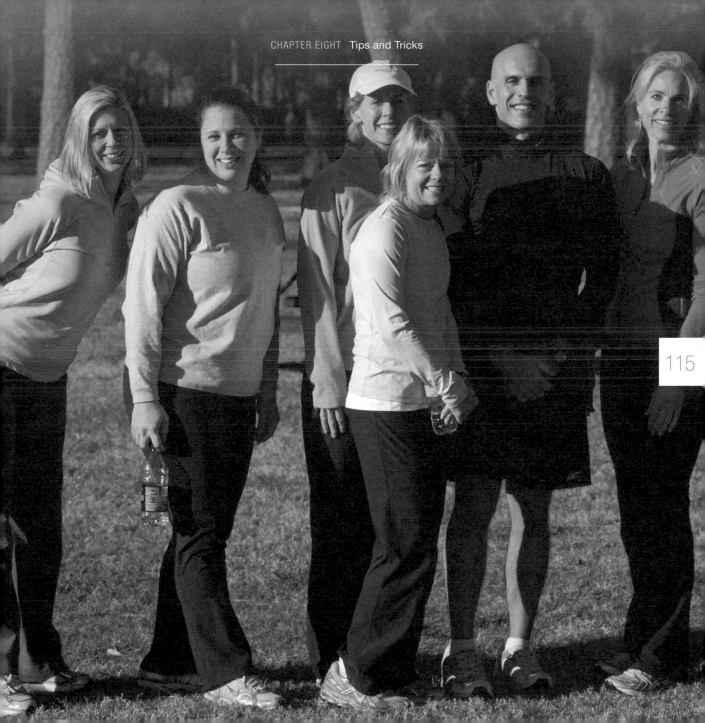

115

Appendices

FOODS WE LIKE

Most of these foods can be found in Houston at
Rice Epicurean Markets.

BARS:

AdvantEdge Carb Control Nutrition Bars - available at
Kroger, Walgreens; store locator at www.eas.com/products

South Beach Diet Bars - Cinnamon Crème is great! Buy
at Walgreens, Kroger and Fiesta Mart

Detour Lower Sugar Caramel Peanut bar!
Go to http://detourbar.com/

Power Crunch bars - available at 24-Hour Fitness & HEB;
fitness center locator at http://www.24hourfitness.com

think Thin all natural high protein bars - buy at Whole
Foods; see store locator at www.thinkproducts.com/

Atkins bars - store locator at http://www.atkins.com/
Products

Titan protein bar is at Kroger. More information at
http://www.premiernutrition.com/

HEALTHY DRINKS:

Special K ice tea-flavored protein powder mix to add
to your water.

Myoplex Carb Sense (protein) Lite Shakes; comes in
packets; store locator at www.eas.com/products

AdvantEdge shakes; see www.eas.com/products for
store locator

Kellogg's k20 comes in single-serve protein packets,
which you add to a glass or bottle of water; available at
grocery and drug stores

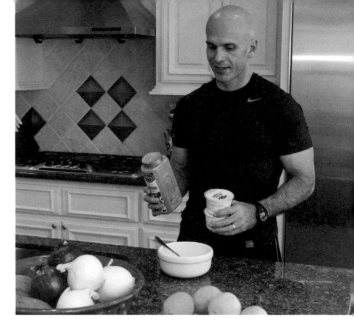

SNACKS:

Mrs. Mays Naturals - cashew crunch; besides COSCO,
locate stores at www.mrsmays.com under "where to buy"

Austin Nut Company has the best pumpkin seeds
available at Central Market

Triscuits with almond butter

"Dr. Kracker" crackers with low-fat cheese are available
at Whole Foods and HEB. Dr. Kracker also makes sweet
ones called Graham Krackers. Dip them in the yogurt for
a sweet treat! Look at http://www.drkracker.com/sales for
other store locations

*Protein Puffs (like Cheetos) and Protein Chips are
great!* For information go to www.nutritionexpress.com/
chef+jays/

Seapoint Farms Dry Roasted Edamame - Besides
Kroger and WalMart, find others at store locator, www.
seapointfarms.com

TrueNorth nut snacks are at Super Target and most food stores like Safeway. Checkout store locator at www.truenorthsnacks.com

Pacific Gold Beef Jerky - For information, call 877-453-7591 or go to www.pacificgoldjerky.com/

DAIRY:

Fagé yogurt - Greek yogurts are all pretty good; watch the sugar added to the fruit ones. Available at Whole Foods and Trader Joe's. See www.traderjoes.com/locations.asp

Breakstone cottage cheese

Smart Balance buttery spread - see product locator at www.smartbalance.com/SBContact.aspx

The Laughing Cow lite cheese - at http://laughingcow.com/ put in your zip code for store locations

SWEETS:

Mrs. Mays Naturals nuts - see www.mrsmays.com for store locations

Walden Farms calorie-free dips - store locator at http://www.waldenfarms.com/

Jello sugar-free pudding and Jello

LaraBar Raw Food Energy bars - Go to www.larabar.com and click on "store" for pull-down menu, then click store locator.

Maya Bars - one of the newest great and natural bars from LaraBar. Available at Whole Foods. See www.larabar.com for other locations

Smucker's Sugar-Free Jelly

VitaMuffins come in apple-berry bran, cran-bran, multi-bran; store locator at www.vitalicious.com

Torani sugar-free syrups - for coffee and other uses; available at Cost Plus World Market; store locator at www.Torani.com

CEREALS/BREADS/CRACKERS:

Fiber One cereal

Grapenuts

"40-30-30 cereal", made by Nutritious Living Hi-Lo, is available at Whole Foods. Go to http://www.wholefoodsmarket.com/stores

"Ezekiel 4:9" organic cereal; for more information go to http://www.foodforlife.com/

Shredded Wheat

Kashi crackers - http://kashi.com/store_finder

Dr. Kracker crackers at Whole Foods, HEB; store locator at http://dr.kracker.com

Alpine Valley Natural Whole Grain bread - see "where to buy" at www.alpinevalleybread.com/index.html

Men's Bread & Women's Bread - store locator at www.frenchmeadow.com/store-locator

Arrowhead Mills oatmeal - store locator at www.pronto.com/

Nature's Path cereal - store locator at www.naturespath.com/

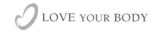

PROTEIN SOURCES

FOOD	SERVING SIZE	GRAMS PROTEIN	CALORIES	GRAMS FAT
95% Lean ground beef	3 oz	21	140	5
Lean roast beef	3 oz	23	147	6
Top sirloin	3 oz	26	156	5
Skinless chicken breast	3 oz	27	140	3
Skinless turkey breast	3 oz	26	115	1
Hot dog	1 each	5	145	13
Pork tenderloin	3 oz	25	171	7
Top loin pork chop	3 oz	25	141	4
Fish	3 oz	21	120	0-4
Canned tuna in water	3 oz	22	99	1
Fresh grilled tuna	3 oz	25	118	1
Flounder or sole	3oz	17	80	1
Salmon	3 oz	21	140	5
Egg	1	6	75	5
Egg whites	2	8	30	0
Nuts	1 oz	7	165	13
Legumes	1 cup	15	225	1

FOOD	SERVING SIZE	GRAMS PROTEIN	CALORIES	GRAMS FAT
Tofu	1 cup	20	176	11
Tempeh (soybeans)	1 cup	31	320	18
Peanut butter	2 tablespoons	8	188	16
Hummus	½ cup	9	204	12
Roasted soybeans	1 oz	11	126	6
Edamame	1 cup	17	189	8
Skim milk	1 cup	12	90	0
Soy milk	1 cup	7	81	4
Nonfat yogurt	1 cup	14	137	0
Grated parmesan cheese	1 oz	12	129	9
Swiss cheese	1 oz	8	107	8
Part-skim mozzarella	1 oz	7	72	4
American cheese	1 oz	6	106	9
Soft goat cheese	1 oz	6	103	8
Fat-free cottage cheese	½ cup	12	62	0
1% Fat cottage cheese	½ cup	14	81	1

Lynn Grieger, RD, CDE
Health, Food and Fitness coach

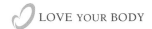

HELPFUL INFO

SUPPORT: WEBSITES

Kaysnaturals.com

Chefjays.com

Realage.com

www.LynnGrieger.com

HELPFUL INFORMATION

Books:

YOU On a Diet by Michael F. Roizen, M.D., & Mehmet C. Oz., M.D.

Copyright 2006; Simon & Schuster, ISBN: 978-0-7432-9154-1

YOU Staying Young: The Owner's Manual for Extending Your Warranty by Michael F. Roizen, M.D., & Mehmet C. Oz., M.D., Copyright 2007; Simon & Schuster, ISBN: 978-0-7432-9256-6

YOU The Owner's Manual Updated and Expanded by Michael F. Roizen, M.D., & Mehmet C. Oz., M.D., Copyright 2008; HarperCollins, ISBN: 978-0-06-1473678.

Body For Life for Women: A Woman's Plan for Physical and Mental Transformation by Pamela Peeke, M.D., Copyright 2005; Foreword by Cindy Crawford; Macmillan Publisher, ISBN: 978-1-59397-643-7.

Gear:

lululemon athletica – you know that v-necks make you look 10 lbs thinner. They make a great jacket with air vents (perfect for warmer days when you want to be covered)

Nike shorts

Nike Medicine Balls

Stroops Resistance Bands

www.academy.com

Finding a Trainer - What to look for:

1. Must be nationally certified – Two certification groups are: American College of Sports Medicine, www.acsm.org; and National Strength and Conditioning Association, www.nsca-lift.org

2. Watch him or her train: – Do you like their style? Are the clients having fun while training? Does he or she change up their routines?

3. Talk to his or her clients – get recommendations!

Love Your Body Fitness Boot Camps information:

www.LoveYourBodyFitness.com

FOOD JOURNAL

Download at www.LoveYourBodyFitness.com

Date: _____			
MEAL	**Time of day**	**What did you eat?**	**Did you have protein? What was your mood?**
#1 (wake up)			
#2			
#3			
#4			
#5			
#6 (2-3 hours prior to bed)			

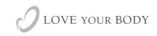

EXERCISE JOURNAL

Download at www.LoveYourBodyFitness.com

Basic Eight	What exercise?	No. of sets/reps
Chest		
Shoulder		
Back		
Biceps		
Triceps		
Legs		
Abs		
Lower Back		
Cardio		

124

APPENDICES

BASIC EIGHT WALLET CARDS

GYM

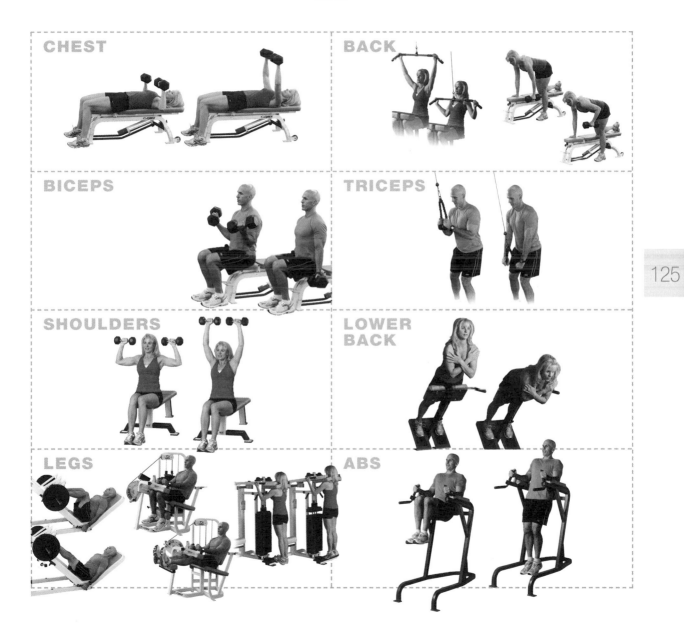

CHEST

BACK

BICEPS

TRICEPS

SHOULDERS

LOWER BACK

LEGS

ABS

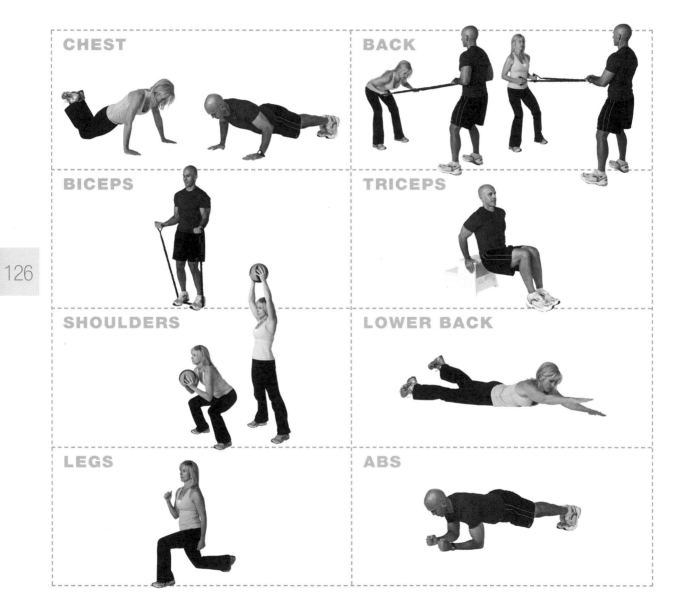

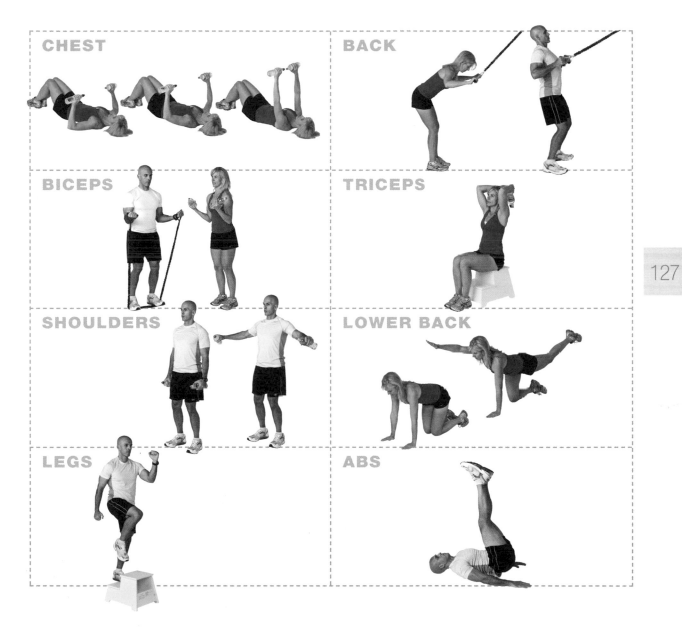

ABOUT THE AUTHORS

VINCE GRBIC, M.ED., C.S.C.S.

Vince has more than 20 years of fitness experience. His philosophy is simple: Always be in motion and make sure you are having fun, so you'll be diligent about your fitness. Vince is currently a personal trainer and has worked as lead trainer in many boot camp and weight-loss programs. He has trained all fitness levels and ages. He was also lead trainer for the George Foreman Walking Videos and fitness director for Red Abdominal exerciser. He has a master's of education degree in health and exercise-related fitness from the University of Houston. He is a professional member and Certified Strength and Conditioning Specialist with the National Strength and Conditioning Association and a professional member and Certified Health Fitness Specialist with the American College of Sports Medicine.

BETHANY HUGHES

Bethany is the co-founder of Love Your Body Fitness Boot Camp. She is a reformed dieter, and living proof that it is possible to love your body — no matter how old you are when you start.

She graduated from Baylor University with a B.A. in Museum Studies and French and a minor in Public Relations. After working in the art world in Dallas, she and her husband moved to Poland, London and now reside in Houston with their two children.

For lots more tips on how to turn any of our exercises into games for a group, check out the website www.loveyourbodyfitness.com. You'll find lots of variations to keep these basic movements interesting and challenging, and we're there for support and to answer any questions you might have.